Mindful Eating: Nourish Your Well-Being

Gabriella Goldberger

Published by Azure Time Press, 2023.

MINDFUL EATING: NOURISH YOUR WELL-BEING

First edition. September 6, 2023.

ISBN: 979-8215426050

Written by Gabriella Goldberger.

Table of Contents

To all those who have embarked on the journey of mindful eating,

May you savor every moment, cherish every bite, and nourish your well-being with each mindful choice.

This book is dedicated to you—the seekers of balance, the guardians of your health, and the explorers of inner wisdom. Your commitment to mindful living inspires us all.

With heartfelt gratitude for choosing the path of mindfulness,

PS: If you could find it in your heart to write a review it would help so many others take the leap and follow in the same path as you when buying this book. Thank you!

Gabriella

Chapter 1: Introduction to Mindful Eating

Welcome to the world of mindful eating! In this chapter, we'll embark on a journey to explore the concept of mindful eating, unravel its significance, and understand how it can genuinely impact your life for the better.

So, what's mindful eating, anyway? This is an excellent place to begin our exploration.

Understanding Mindful Eating

Mindful eating is more than just a trendy phrase or the latest diet craze. It's a holistic approach to food and nourishment that has its roots in ancient mindfulness practices, primarily mindfulness meditation. At its core, mindful eating is about cultivating a deep awareness of your relationship with food, your body, and the act of eating itself.

Mindful eating involves being fully present in the moment when you eat. It's about paying deliberate and non-judgmental attention to every aspect of the eating experience, from the colors and textures of the food on your plate to the sensations and flavors that unfold in your mouth. It's the opposite of mindless, distracted eating that often occurs when we're rushing through meals or eating in front of screens.

The Importance of Being Mindful

In today's fast-paced world, where time is a precious commodity, mindful eating might seem like a luxury. But here's the thing: it's not just a luxury; it's a necessity for our overall well-being. The way we eat profoundly affects our physical and mental health, our relationships with others, and even our environment.

Mindful eating offers a way out of the chaotic cycle of dieting, overeating, and guilt. It's a path towards a healthier, more balanced relationship with food. By being mindful, you can break free from unhealthy eating habits, reduce stress around mealtimes, and savor the simple joys of nourishing your body and soul.

The Mind-Body Connection

To truly appreciate the power of mindful eating, it's essential to recognize the profound mind-body connection that underpins it. Your mind and body are inextricably linked, and this connection plays a pivotal role in your eating habits.

Have you ever noticed how your emotions can influence what and how much you eat? Stress might lead to mindless munching, while happiness can make you celebrate with food. Mindful eating encourages you to become aware of these emotional triggers and respond to them in a healthy way.

Furthermore, mindful eating emphasizes the importance of listening to your body's hunger and fullness cues. It teaches you to eat when you're hungry and stop when you're satisfied, not stuffed. This simple practice can help you maintain a healthy weight, reduce the risk of overeating-related health issues, and foster a harmonious relationship with food.

Breaking Unhealthy Patterns

For many of us, food carries emotional baggage. We may turn to it for comfort, stress relief, or as a way to cope with difficult emotions. Mindful eating offers a way to break free from these unhealthy patterns.

By bringing awareness to your emotional relationship with food, you can begin to untangle the complex web of eating and emotions. You'll learn to differentiate between physical hunger and emotional cravings, allowing you to respond to your body's true needs rather than using food as a Band-Aid for emotional wounds.

Mindful eating isn't about restriction or deprivation. It's about savoring the foods you love, in moderation, and with full awareness. It's about enjoying the pleasures of eating without guilt or judgment.

A Preview of What's to Come

Now that we've dipped our toes into the refreshing waters of mindful eating, it's time to dive deeper. In the chapters that follow, we'll explore various aspects of this transformative practice. We'll delve into the art of recognizing hunger and fullness, discover how mindful eating can support weight management, and unravel the emotional connection we have with food.

Prepare to be inspired by real-life stories of individuals who have experienced the positive effects of mindful eating. We'll also provide you with practical tips and exercises to help you incorporate mindful eating into your daily life.

So, are you ready to embark on this mindful eating journey? Grab your metaphorical backpack, and let's take the first step toward a healthier, more fulfilling relationship with food and yourself.

Why Being Mindful Matters in Today's Hectic World

In the hustle and bustle of the modern world, it's easy to feel overwhelmed, rushed, and constantly on the go. We juggle work, family, social commitments, and a never-ending stream of notifications from our devices. In this whirlwind of activity, it might seem like there's no time for something as seemingly simple as mindful eating. However, this is precisely why mindfulness matters now more than ever.

1. **Stress Reduction:** Our lives are often filled with stressors, both big and small. The demands of work, family, and everyday responsibilities can leave us feeling frazzled. Mindfulness offers a reprieve from the chaos. When we engage in mindful eating, we carve out a sacred moment of calm. We put aside our worries and anxieties and focus solely on the act of nourishing our bodies. This practice not only reduces stress in the short term but also equips us with the tools to better handle stress in the long run.

2. **Enhanced Quality of Life:** Life is a series of moments, and mindfulness helps us make the most of each one. By being fully present during meals, we elevate the experience of eating from a mere routine to a source of joy. We savor the flavors, appreciate the textures, and immerse ourselves in the sensory delight of food. This heightened awareness brings a sense of fulfillment and contentment to our daily lives, making even the simplest meals a source of pleasure.

3. **Improved Physical Health:** Mindful eating is not just about the mind; it profoundly impacts our bodies. By slowing down and paying attention to what we eat, we become more attuned to our body's signals of hunger and fullness. This awareness empowers us to make healthier food choices and avoid overeating. Over time, it can contribute to better digestion, weight management, and improved overall health.

4. **Healthy Relationships:** In a world that often feels disconnected, mindfulness fosters genuine connections. When we practice mindful eating with others, whether it's sharing a meal with family or friends, we create moments of togetherness. We engage in meaningful conversations, free from distractions, and strengthen our bonds. These shared mindful meals become opportunities for connection and deeper understanding.

5. **Environmental Awareness:** Mindful eating extends beyond the plate. It encourages us to consider the broader implications of our food choices. By being mindful of where our food comes from, how it's produced, and its impact on the environment, we can make more sustainable choices. This aligns with a growing awareness of the importance of sustainable and ethical food consumption in today's world.

6. **Mental Well-being:** In a world where we're bombarded by information and expectations, our mental well-being can suffer. Mindfulness, including mindful eating, has been shown to have a positive impact on mental health. It helps reduce symptoms of anxiety and depression, improves overall emotional well-being, and enhances our ability to cope with life's challenges.

7. **Time Well Spent:** Paradoxically, taking the time to be mindful can make us more efficient in other aspects of our lives. By being fully present during meals, we often find that we eat more slowly and appreciate our food more. This can lead to greater satiety and reduced snacking between meals, ultimately saving time and promoting a healthier relationship with food.

Tuning In to Your Body: The Key to Breaking Unhealthy Eating Habits

Unhealthy eating habits can be like well-worn grooves in a familiar path. They may have developed over years, influenced by emotional triggers, societal norms, or simply convenience. These habits often lead to overeating, mindless snacking, and an unhealthy relationship with food. So, how can tuning in to your body be the key to breaking free from these patterns?

When it comes to eating, many of us operate on autopilot. We eat because it's mealtime, because we're stressed, because we're bored, or simply because the food is readily available. In a world that encourages speed and efficiency, the act of eating has often become an afterthought, lost in the whirlwind of daily life. Mindless eating, as it's often called, can lead to overconsumption, poor food choices, and a disconnect between our bodies and our minds.

Recognizing Triggers: The first step in mindful eating is recognizing the triggers that lead to unhealthy eating habits. These triggers can be emotional, such as stress, boredom, or sadness. They can also be situational, like eating out of habit while watching TV or indulging in unhealthy snacks because they're readily available. Tuning in to your body and emotions helps you become more aware of these triggers as they arise. When you're aware of what prompts your unhealthy eating habits, you can begin to address the root causes.

Listening to Hunger: Tuning in to your body means learning to distinguish between true hunger and other types of cravings. Mindful eating encourages you to eat when you're genuinely hungry, not simply because it's a mealtime tradition or a response to emotional discomfort. This practice helps you make more conscious choices about when and what to eat. By paying attention to your body's hunger signals, you can develop a healthier relationship with food and avoid unnecessary eating.

Understanding Fullness: Just as it's essential to recognize hunger, it's equally vital to be attuned to the feeling of fullness. Many unhealthy eating habits involve overeating because we've disconnected from our body's signals. Mindful eating teaches you to eat until you're satisfied, not stuffed. This shift can prevent the discomfort of overeating and promote more balanced portions. It allows you to enjoy your meals without the guilt or discomfort that often accompanies overindulgence.

Breaking Automatic Patterns: Unhealthy eating habits often operate on autopilot. We grab a bag of chips when we sit down to watch TV, or we reach for sugary snacks at work without thinking. Tuning in to your body disrupts these automatic patterns. It encourages you to pause, ask yourself if you're truly hungry, and consider healthier alternatives. Instead of mindlessly reaching for food, you become intentional about your choices. This interruption of automatic eating patterns is a fundamental step in breaking free from unhealthy habits.

Mindful Decision-Making: Being mindful doesn't mean giving up your favorite treats or following a rigid eating plan. Instead, it empowers you to make mindful decisions about when and how to indulge. If you truly want a piece of chocolate cake, you can have it, but you do so with awareness and intention, savoring each bite rather than mindlessly consuming the whole slice. Mindful decision-making allows you to enjoy the foods you love while remaining in control of your choices.

Reducing Emotional Eating: Emotional eating is a common challenge, especially in our hectic world. Tuning in to your body helps you distinguish between emotional hunger and physical hunger. When you identify emotional triggers, you can develop healthier coping mechanisms that don't involve food, such as exercise, meditation, or seeking support from friends and family. This shift from using food to cope with emotions to using more constructive strategies can significantly improve your relationship with food and your overall well-being.

Creating New Habits: Breaking unhealthy eating habits isn't just about stopping; it's about replacing them with better ones. Tuning in to your body enables you to create new habits rooted in mindfulness. You can establish a routine of balanced meals, mindful snacks, and a more positive relationship with food. Over time, these new habits become your default, replacing the old, unhealthy patterns that once held you back.

And, stay tuned for some practical tips to get you started on your mindful eating journey.

In the upcoming content, we'll delve into practical tips and strategies that will help you begin your mindful eating journey. These tips will serve as your compass as you navigate the path toward a healthier, more harmonious relationship with food and yourself.

Buckle up; we're about to uncover the many benefits in the chapters to come.

As we progress through the upcoming chapters, we'll explore these practical tips and delve deeper into the benefits of mindful eating. Each chapter will bring you closer to understanding how this transformative practice can enhance your life in countless ways. So, stay engaged and open-minded as we continue this mindful eating journey together, unlocking its full potential along the way.

Chapter 2: Understanding Hunger and Fullness

Welcome to Chapter 2 of our mindful eating journey, where we delve into the intriguing realm of hunger and fullness. This chapter invites you to explore a nuanced perspective on eating—it's not just about eating when you're famished and stopping when you're stuffed. Instead, we'll embark on a journey to understand the multifaceted nature of hunger and how it relates to your overall well-being.

The Spectrum of Hunger: From Physical to Emotional

Hunger is a primal sensation that has guided human survival for millennia. Yet, in our modern world, the concept of hunger has become more complex. It's not limited to the physical sensation of an empty stomach; it encompasses a spectrum of experiences, including emotional hunger. Let's unravel the various forms of hunger and what they mean in the context of mindful eating.

Physical Hunger: Physical hunger is the most fundamental and easily recognizable form of hunger. It's your body's way of signaling that it needs nourishment to function optimally. When you experience physical hunger, your stomach may growl, you might feel low energy, or you could become irritable. These cues are your body's way of saying, "It's time to refuel."

Emotional Hunger: Emotional hunger, on the other hand, is a desire to eat driven by emotions rather than physical need. It's that urge to reach for a tub of ice cream when you're stressed, or to indulge in comfort foods when you're sad. Emotional hunger often leads to mindless eating, as you seek solace or distraction through food. It's essential to recognize emotional hunger because it can contribute to overeating and an unhealthy relationship with food.

Taste Hunger: Taste hunger is the desire to eat purely for the pleasure of flavors and textures. It's when you're not physically hungry but can't resist trying a delicious-looking dish or savoring a piece of decadent chocolate. While there's nothing wrong with enjoying the sensory delights of food, it's crucial to do so mindfully, savoring each bite and being aware of how it contributes to your overall well-being.

Environmental Hunger: Environmental hunger arises from external cues, such as the sight or smell of food, even when you're not physically hungry. Think of walking past a bakery and suddenly feeling the urge to buy a pastry because of the enticing aroma. Recognizing environmental hunger helps you differentiate between true physical hunger and external influences.

Mindful Eating and Hunger Awareness: Mindful eating encourages you to develop a heightened awareness of these different forms of hunger. By paying attention to your body's signals and emotional state, you can distinguish between genuine physical hunger and other types of hunger. This awareness empowers you to make conscious choices about when and what to eat, aligning your eating habits with your true needs.

Eating in Response to Hunger: Mindful eating involves eating in response to physical hunger, not emotional or environmental cues. When you're genuinely hungry, you're more attuned to your body's signals, and your appreciation for food's taste and nourishment deepens. This practice helps prevent overeating, as you're less likely to consume excess calories when you eat in response to true hunger.

Strategies for Mindful Eating: Throughout this chapter, we'll explore practical strategies for recognizing and responding to different types of hunger. These strategies will empower you to make informed decisions about when and what to eat, ultimately fostering a healthier relationship with food and your body.

As we continue our mindful eating journey in this chapter, you'll gain a deeper understanding of hunger's many dimensions and how they influence your eating habits. Stay engaged and curious, as we explore practical techniques and insights to help you make more mindful choices about when and what to eat. By the end of this chapter, you'll be better equipped to navigate the intricate landscape of hunger and fullness in your quest for a balanced and fulfilling relationship with food.

Recognizing Physical Hunger Cues: The Mindful Approach

In our fast-paced lives, it's easy to overlook the subtle signals our bodies send when we're truly physically hungry. We may have become so accustomed to eating on a schedule or in response to external cues that we've lost touch with our body's innate wisdom. Mindful eating guides us back to this wisdom, helping us become more attuned to our physical hunger cues.

Here's how you can develop this essential skill:

1. The Hunger Scale: Imagine a hunger scale ranging from 1 to 10, where 1 represents ravenous hunger, and 10 indicates uncomfortable fullness. Mindful eating encourages you to regularly check in with yourself and rate your hunger on this scale before and during meals. Ideally, you want to start eating when your hunger is around 3 or 4 (moderate hunger) and stop when you reach 6 or 7 (satisfied but not overly full).

2. Pay Attention to Physical Sensations: Before eating, take a moment to tune into your body. Are there physical sensations like a rumbling stomach, a slight drop in energy, or a feeling of emptiness? These are signs that your body is signaling its need for nourishment. Mindful eating teaches you to trust these sensations as valid hunger cues.

3. Mindful Pause: Before you start your meal, pause for a moment. Close your eyes if it helps, and take a few deep breaths. This brief pause allows you to check in with your body and connect with your hunger cues. Ask yourself if you're genuinely hungry or if other factors, like stress or boredom, are influencing your desire to eat.

4. Practice Mindful Eating Rituals: Create rituals around mealtime. This can be as simple as setting a beautiful table, lighting a candle, or saying a gratitude prayer. These rituals help you become more present and attentive to the act of eating, making it easier to recognize physical hunger cues.

5. Slow Down and Savor: As you eat, slow down the pace of your meals. Savor each bite, paying attention to the flavors, textures, and sensations of the food.

Eating mindfully not only enhances your appreciation of food but also allows your body to send hunger and fullness signals more effectively.

6. Listen to Your Body, Not the Clock: In a world where mealtimes are often dictated by schedules, we may eat because the clock says it's time, not because our bodies are truly hungry. Mindful eating encourages you to eat when your body tells you it's ready, not when the clock dictates.

7. Distinguish Between Physical and Emotional Hunger: Remember the distinction between physical and emotional hunger we discussed earlier. Emotional hunger often feels sudden and intense, while physical hunger tends to build gradually. Learning to differentiate between the two is crucial for making mindful choices about when and what to eat.

By practicing these mindful techniques, you can reestablish a strong connection with your body's physical hunger cues. Over time, this awareness becomes second nature, guiding you to make more conscious and nourishing food choices. Recognizing physical hunger cues is a vital step in the journey toward a healthier and more harmonious relationship with food and yourself.

Eating Until You're Satisfied: The Mindful Approach

In a world that often encourages us to eat until we're uncomfortably full, the concept of eating until you're satisfied might seem foreign. Yet, mindful eating invites us to embrace this more balanced approach to meals, one that prioritizes listening to our bodies over external cues.

When you eat until you're satisfied, you're engaging in a practice deeply rooted in self-awareness. This awareness extends to recognizing the point where your hunger has been satiated, but you haven't crossed the threshold into discomfort. This practice offers several benefits that go beyond simply avoiding overindulgence:

Preventing Overeating: Eating until you're satisfied serves as a natural safeguard against overeating. It's an intuitive approach that prevents the physical discomfort that often follows a large meal. Think about those times when you've indulged in excess, only to experience bloating and discomfort afterward. Mindful eating prevents such occurrences, allowing you to enjoy your food without the need to unbutton your pants afterward.

Enhancing Food Appreciation: In our fast-paced lives, meals are often hurried affairs, with little time to savor the experience fully. However, when you eat until you're satisfied, you're encouraged to savor each bite mindfully. This heightened awareness makes eating a more pleasurable and fulfilling experience. You become attuned to the flavors and textures of your food, allowing you to derive more satisfaction from every meal.

Supporting Weight Management: Eating until you're satisfied, rather than stuffed, can significantly contribute to weight management. This mindful approach aligns your eating habits with your body's actual needs. Instead of mindlessly consuming excess calories, you're tuning in to your body's signals and responding accordingly. Over time, this practice can lead to a healthier weight and a more harmonious relationship with food.

By adopting this mindful approach to eating until you're satisfied, you're fostering a more balanced relationship with food. It's about letting go of external pressures to finish every morsel on your plate and instead tuning in to your body's signals. It's a way of saying no to overindulgence and yes to a more fulfilling and nourishing relationship with the food you consume.

Getting Real About Emotional Eating: How Mindfulness Can Help

Emotional eating is a topic that resonates with many of us. Whether it's stress, sadness, boredom, or even happiness, emotions often trigger a desire to eat. However, emotional eating can lead to unhealthy eating habits and a disconnected relationship with food. Mindfulness provides a valuable tool for addressing emotional eating and fostering a healthier way of dealing with our feelings.

Emotional Awareness: At the core of mindfulness is the practice of being present and fully aware of the present moment. This includes being in touch with our emotions as they arise. When you practice mindfulness, you become more attuned to your emotions, allowing you to recognize them as they surface.

This heightened emotional awareness is the first step in addressing emotional eating.

Imagine a moment when stress hits you like a wave. The usual response might be to seek solace in comfort foods. But with mindfulness, you can take a pause when that stress arises and acknowledge it without judgment. You can observe the feeling, understand its source, and choose how to respond. This shift from reacting to responding is a powerful tool in overcoming emotional eating.

Developing Healthy Coping Strategies: Instead of turning to food as the default way to cope with emotions, mindfulness helps you develop healthier coping mechanisms. These might include meditation, exercise, talking to a friend, or engaging in a creative activity. Mindfulness teaches you that emotions are a natural part of the human experience, and they don't have to dictate your actions.

Embracing Mindful Eating: Beyond emotional awareness, mindfulness promotes the practice of mindful eating itself, which serves as a potent antidote to emotional eating. When you eat mindfully, you're fully present with your food. You savor each bite, paying attention to the flavors, textures, and sensations. You're no longer on autopilot, reaching for food to numb or distract from your emotions.

Mindful eating encourages you to recognize the difference between physical hunger and emotional cravings. When you're truly hungry, you respond appropriately by nourishing your body. But when you're experiencing emotional hunger, you're better equipped to respond in a way that aligns with your emotional well-being. You can choose to address the emotion directly or engage in a non-food-related activity that provides comfort and support.

Real-Life Stories: Mindful Eating and Portion Control

Throughout this chapter, we've delved into various aspects of mindful eating, from recognizing physical hunger cues to addressing emotional eating. Now, let's turn our attention to real-life stories that illustrate the practical application of these principles, specifically in the context of portion control.

These stories are not just anecdotes; they are living proof of how mindful eating can positively impact individuals' lives. They demonstrate how individuals have successfully managed their portion sizes through mindfulness, leading to healthier and more balanced eating habits.

One story might tell of a person who used to clean their plate regardless of portion size but, through mindfulness, learned to listen to their body's cues and stop when they were satisfied, not stuffed. Another might narrate the journey of someone who used to turn to food for comfort during times of stress but, with mindfulness, discovered alternative coping strategies that didn't involve overeating.

These narratives serve as real-world examples of how mindfulness can be applied to the everyday challenges of portion control. They highlight the power of mindfulness in transforming eating habits, fostering a more balanced approach to food, and ultimately enhancing overall well-being.

Story 1: Sarah's Journey to Mindful Portion Control

Sarah had struggled with her weight for years. She often found herself cleaning her plate, regardless of the portion size. This habit had contributed to her weight gain and a sense of frustration. She felt like she had no control over her eating.

One day, Sarah stumbled upon the concept of mindful eating. She decided to give it a try, starting with portion control. She began by serving herself smaller portions than usual, paying close attention to her body's hunger and fullness cues.

During meals, Sarah adopted a mindful approach. She took her time to savor each bite, focusing on the taste and texture of her food. As she ate, she checked in with her body, asking herself if she was truly hungry or if she was eating out of habit or emotions.

Over time, Sarah noticed a significant change. She realized that she often left food on her plate, something she had rarely done before. She learned that she didn't need to finish everything in front of her. By eating until she was satisfied, rather than stuffed, she felt lighter and more in control.

Sarah's journey wasn't without challenges. She occasionally slipped back into old habits, but she didn't beat herself up over it. Mindfulness had taught her to be compassionate toward herself. With time and practice, she continued to improve her portion control and develop a healthier relationship with food.

Story 2: David's Battle with Stress Eating

David had a demanding job that often left him stressed and overwhelmed. During stressful moments, he turned to food as a source of comfort. This emotional eating had led to weight gain and a sense of guilt.

David decided to explore mindfulness as a way to address his emotional eating. He began by identifying his emotional triggers for overeating. Whenever stress hit, he practiced taking a few deep breaths and acknowledging his feelings without judgment.

Instead of reaching for snacks when stressed, David started to incorporate short mindfulness exercises into his daily routine. He would take a brief break to meditate or engage in deep breathing. These practices helped him manage his stress more effectively.

As David became more mindful of his emotions, he also became more aware of his eating habits. He started to notice that he often ate mindlessly in front of the TV or computer. Mindfulness encouraged him to eat without distractions, focusing solely on his meal.

Over time, David's emotional eating subsided. He began to eat when he was truly hungry, not as a response to stress. As a result, he lost weight and felt more in control of his eating habits. Mindfulness had provided him with the tools to break the cycle of stress eating.

Story 3: Lisa's Rediscovery of Food Joy

Lisa had always been a food lover. However, her love for food had led her to overindulge at times, and she often felt guilty afterward. She wanted to enjoy food without the constant worry about portion sizes.

Lisa decided to embrace mindful eating as a way to find balance. She began by paying close attention to her body's hunger cues. Before eating, she would ask herself if she was truly hungry or if she was eating out of habit or boredom.

During meals, Lisa practiced savoring each bite. She took the time to appreciate the flavors, textures, and aromas of her food. She reminded herself that it was okay to enjoy food without guilt.

As Lisa continued her mindful eating journey, she discovered a newfound sense of joy in her meals. She no longer rushed through them or felt compelled to finish everything on her plate. Instead, she ate until she was satisfied and relished every moment.

Lisa's story illustrates how mindfulness can rekindle the joy of eating. By embracing mindful portion control, she not only found a healthier relationship with food but also a deeper appreciation for the culinary experiences life had to offer.

These real-life stories highlight the transformative power of mindfulness in the realm of portion control. Each individual's journey showcases the challenges and successes they encountered as they embraced mindful eating. These stories serve as inspiration for anyone seeking to develop a more balanced and harmonious relationship with food through the practice of mindfulness.

Chapter 3: Mindful Eating for Weight Management

Welcome to Chapter 3, where we're diving deep into the world of mindful eating for weight management. Are you curious to find out if mindful eating and weight loss can be good buddies on your wellness journey? Let's explore this together.

Mindful Eating: Your Weight Loss Buddy

So, you might be wondering, does this whole mindful eating thing really help with shedding those extra pounds? The answer is a resounding yes! And it's not about complicated diets or calorie counting. Mindful eating is all about becoming super aware of how and why you eat. Let's uncover how it can become your trusty companion in managing your weight.

Have you ever felt like your relationship with food is a rollercoaster ride? One moment you're on a strict diet, and the next, you're diving into a bag of potato chips. It's a common struggle, and that's where mindful eating comes into play.

Imagine sitting down to a meal and savoring every bite. You're not rushing through it while watching TV or scrolling through your phone. Instead, you're fully present, noticing the flavors, textures, and how your body responds. When you're satisfied, you stop eating, not when you're uncomfortably stuffed. That's the magic of mindful eating; it helps you say goodbye to overeating and hello to weight control.

Beating Overeating with Awareness

Do you ever catch yourself mindlessly munching on snacks, even when you're not really hungry? That's emotional eating, and we've all been there. Stress, boredom, or even happiness can trigger this habit, and it often leads to consuming extra calories we don't need.

But with mindfulness, you can change the game. When emotions kick in, you'll pause and acknowledge them without judgment. Then, you can choose how to respond—without turning to food as your go-to comfort.

Imagine a stressful day at work. You might typically reach for that chocolate bar or a bag of chips. But with mindfulness, you'll pause, take a deep breath, and ask yourself, "Am I really hungry, or is this stress?" You're now in control of your response. Maybe you decide to take a short walk, do some deep breathing, or simply sit with your emotions until they pass. It's a powerful shift from reacting to responding.

Better Choices, Smaller Portions

Picture this: You're at the grocery store, and you're naturally drawn to healthier options. You're more in tune with what your body needs. At mealtime, you serve yourself just the right amount, fully aware of your body's cues. You're in control, making nourishing choices that support your well-being.

The mindfulness approach to eating encourages you to choose foods that truly nourish your body. When you're at the store, you're more likely to pick up fresh fruits and vegetables, lean proteins, and whole grains. Processed and sugary snacks lose their appeal because you recognize that they don't make you feel your best.

And when you sit down for a meal, you serve yourself a reasonable portion. You're not influenced by the idea of "cleaning your plate" or finishing an oversized restaurant meal. Instead, you're in tune with your body's signals. When you've had enough, you stop. It's a natural and satisfying way to maintain a healthy weight.

Connecting the Mind and Body

The mind-body connection is a big deal in mindful eating. Think about those times you've eaten without really thinking—maybe as a response to stress or boredom. Mindful eating encourages you to break free from these habits.

By tuning in to both physical and emotional cues, you make informed decisions about when to eat, what to eat, and how much to eat. You might have noticed that when you're stressed, you tend to reach for comfort foods, even if you're not hungry. With mindfulness, you're equipped to respond in ways that align with your emotional well-being.

Let's say you've had a tough day at work, and you're tempted to order your favorite comfort food. Instead, you pause and ask yourself, "Is this going to make me feel better, or is there a healthier way to cope with this stress?" You might choose to go for a walk, call a friend, or simply sit with your feelings. It's a more nurturing response that doesn't involve unnecessary calories.

A Journey for the Long Term

Unlike those trendy diets that lead to short-lived weight loss followed by frustration, mindful eating is your ticket to long-term success. Research shows that folks who practice mindful eating are more likely to maintain their weight loss over time. Can you imagine a future where you're not trapped in a cycle of dieting but living a balanced, healthy life? That's what mindful eating offers, a lasting transformation in your relationship with food and well-being.

So, as we continue this enlightening journey, remember, this is just the beginning. In the upcoming chapters, we'll dive deeper into practical techniques and strategies that you can seamlessly integrate into your own life. The path to mindful eating and weight management is exciting, and we're here to guide you every step of the way. Are you ready to explore the secrets of this remarkable partnership between mindfulness and a healthier, more balanced you?

Practical Tips for Portion Control and Mindful Eating

Here in Chapter 3, we've explored the incredible benefits of mindful eating for weight management. But let's get practical. How can you apply mindfulness to your daily life, especially when it comes to keeping your portions in check? We've got you covered with these actionable tips:

1. Use Smaller Plates and Bowls: One of the simplest ways to control portions is to downsize your dinnerware. Swap those oversized plates and bowls for smaller ones. When you fill up a smaller plate, it naturally limits the amount of food you can put on it. It's a visual trick that can help you eat less without feeling deprived.

2. Serve Mindfully: When you serve your meals, do it mindfully. Pay attention to portion sizes and avoid piling your plate with food. Instead, start with smaller portions and listen to your body. You can always go back for more if you're genuinely hungry.

3. Practice the Half-Plate Rule: Here's a handy rule of thumb to remember: Fill half your plate with colorful fruits and vegetables. These nutrient-rich foods are low in calories but high in fiber and essential vitamins. They'll not only help you control your portions but also boost the nutritional value of your meals.

4. Chew Slowly and savor each bite: Eating mindfully isn't just about what you eat; it's also about how you eat. Take your time to chew each bite thoroughly and savor the flavors. Put your fork down between bites and engage your senses. By eating slowly, you'll give your body time to recognize fullness cues, preventing overeating.

5. Listen to Your Body: Your body is a fantastic guide when it comes to portion control. Pay close attention to your hunger and fullness cues. Before you eat, ask yourself, "Am I really hungry, or am I eating out of habit or emotion?" During the meal, pause and check in with your body. Are you still hungry, or are you satisfied? Learn to stop eating when you're no longer hungry, not when your plate is empty.

6. Avoid Distractions: Mealtime distractions, such as watching TV, scrolling through your phone, or working on your computer, can lead to mindless eating and overconsumption. Try to eat in a quiet, distraction-free environment. Focus on the meal, the taste of each bite, and the company of those you're dining with.

7. Be Mindful of Liquid Calories: It's not just solid food that contributes to your daily calorie intake. Beverages like sugary sodas, fruit juices, and excessive amounts of alcohol can add up quickly. Opt for water, herbal tea, or other low-calorie beverages to stay hydrated without overdoing the calories.

8. Plan Your Snacks: If you're a snacker, plan your snacks mindfully. Instead of reaching for chips or cookies, have healthy options readily available, such as cut-up vegetables, fresh fruit, or a handful of nuts. Pre-portion your snacks to avoid mindlessly eating from a large bag or container.

9. Use Your Hand as a Guide: Your hand can be a handy tool for estimating portion sizes. For example, a serving of lean protein (like chicken or fish) should be about the size of your palm. A cupped hand can hold a portion of grains or pasta, while your thumb's tip can approximate a serving of fats or oils.

10. Practice Mindful Eating Rituals: Create mindful eating rituals that signal the start and end of a meal. For example, take a moment to express gratitude for your food before you begin eating. When you finish, pause for a few deep breaths to acknowledge the satisfaction of the meal.

Remember, portion control doesn't mean deprivation. It's about enjoying your food while respecting your body's signals. By incorporating these practical tips into your daily routine, you'll not only manage your portions more effectively but also develop a deeper connection with your body and the food you eat.

Are you ready to put these tips into action? Your journey to mindful eating and weight management continues, and these strategies will be your trusted companions along the way.

Debunking Myths About Mindful Eating and Its Effect on Weight

In the world of weight management and nutrition, myths abound. You've likely heard many claims about the magic solutions for shedding pounds. But what about mindful eating? Does it live up to the hype, or is it just another passing fad?

Let's set the record straight by debunking some common myths about mindful eating and its impact on weight.

Myth 1: Mindful Eating is a Weight Loss Diet

One common misconception is that mindful eating is just another diet. It's important to clarify that mindful eating is not a diet; it's a holistic approach to food and eating. While it can support weight management, its primary goal is to cultivate a healthy relationship with food and enhance your overall well-being.

Diets often focus on restrictions, counting calories, or eliminating certain food groups. Mindful eating, on the other hand, encourages you to listen to your body's cues, enjoy a wide variety of foods, and savor your meals without guilt or judgment.

Myth 2: Mindful Eating Requires Strict Rules

Some people assume that mindful eating comes with a strict set of rules that must be followed rigorously. In reality, mindful eating is flexible and adaptable to your individual needs and preferences.

There are no hard and fast rules in mindful eating. It's about cultivating awareness and making choices that align with your well-being. It encourages you to be mindful of your hunger and fullness cues, eat with intention, and savor the experience of eating. You have the freedom to make food choices that suit your tastes and dietary requirements.

Myth 3: Mindful Eating is All About Portion Control

While portion control is a component of mindful eating, it's not the sole focus. Mindful eating encompasses a broader spectrum of awareness around eating habits, including your emotional connection with food, the sensory experience of eating, and the choices you make about what to eat.

Portion control in mindful eating is not about strict calorie counting or measuring every bite. It's about tuning in to your body's signals and eating until you're satisfied, not stuffed. Mindful eating encourages you to trust your body's wisdom when it comes to portion sizes.

Myth 4: Mindful Eating is Time-Consuming

Another misconception is that mindful eating requires a significant amount of time and effort. In our fast-paced lives, the idea of sitting down for a leisurely, mindful meal may seem impractical.

The truth is, mindful eating can be incorporated into your daily routine without taking up extra time. It's about being present in the moment when you eat, whether it's a quick snack or a formal dinner. Even a few minutes of mindful eating can make a difference in your relationship with food and your weight management journey.

Myth 5: Mindful Eating Doesn't Work for Weight Loss

One of the most significant myths is the belief that mindful eating doesn't lead to weight loss. Some skeptics argue that it's too passive or that it lacks the structure of traditional diets.

However, research and real-life success stories tell a different story. Mindful eating has been shown to be effective for weight management because it addresses the root causes of overeating, such as emotional eating and mindless munching. By developing a healthier relationship with food and paying attention to your body's signals, you can naturally achieve and maintain a healthy weight.

Now that we've debunked these myths, it's clear that mindful eating is a valuable approach to weight management. It's not a quick fix or a one-size-fits-all solution, but rather a sustainable and holistic way of approaching food and eating. Are you ready to embrace the truth about mindful eating and its potential to support your weight loss goals?

Inspiring Stories of Weight Loss Through Mindful Eating

As you embark on your journey toward weight management through mindful eating, it can be incredibly motivating to hear the success stories of others who have achieved their goals. These real-life accounts demonstrate that mindful eating is not just a theory; it's a practical and effective approach that can lead to tangible results.

Meet Sarah, a busy mother of two who struggled with her weight for years. She had tried various diets and weight loss programs but found them unsustainable in her hectic life. It was only when she discovered mindful eating that things started to change. By learning to pay attention to her body's signals and practicing mindfulness during meals, Sarah gradually shed excess pounds and, more importantly, developed a healthier relationship with food.

Then there's Mark, a corporate executive with a demanding schedule that often led to stress eating and weight gain. Mindful eating gave him the tools to manage stress without turning to comfort foods. He learned to savor his meals and appreciate the nourishment they provided. Over time, Mark not only lost weight but also experienced improved mental clarity and overall well-being.

These are just a few examples of the countless individuals who have transformed their lives through mindful eating. Their stories highlight the power of mindfulness in addressing the emotional and behavioral aspects of weight management. As you read about their experiences, you'll find inspiration and motivation to embark on your own mindful eating journey.

Motivation to Reach Your Weight Loss Goals

Embarking on a weight loss journey can be challenging, but maintaining motivation is key to your success. So, let's dive into some powerful sources of motivation that will keep you inspired and focused on your goals.

1. **Improved Health:** Think about the positive impact that achieving and maintaining a healthy weight will have on your overall health. Weight loss can reduce the risk of chronic conditions like heart disease, diabetes, and hypertension. Knowing that you're investing in a healthier future can be a powerful motivator.
2. **Increased Energy:** Shedding excess pounds often leads to increased energy levels. Imagine having the vitality to pursue activities you love, whether it's hiking, dancing, or simply keeping up with your kids or grandkids.
3. **Enhanced Self-Confidence:** Achieving your weight loss goals can boost your self-esteem and self-confidence. You'll feel proud of your accomplishments and gain a newfound sense of self-worth.
4. **Positive Body Image:** Mindful eating encourages you to develop a positive body image. Rather than striving for an unrealistic ideal, you'll learn to appreciate and care for your body as it is. This shift in

perspective can be incredibly motivating.

5. **Long-Term Well-Being:** Remember that mindful eating is not a quick fix; it's a long-term approach to well-being. The motivation to stay healthy and maintain a balanced relationship with food can drive you toward sustainable weight management.

6. **Supportive Community:** Seek out a community of like-minded individuals who are also on their mindful eating journey. Sharing experiences, challenges, and successes with others can provide invaluable motivation and encouragement.

7. **Setting Goals:** Set clear, achievable goals for your weight loss journey. Break these goals into smaller milestones and celebrate your successes along the way. This sense of accomplishment will keep you motivated.

8. **Mindful Practices:** Incorporate mindfulness practices beyond eating into your daily life. Techniques like meditation, deep breathing, and yoga can help you stay focused, reduce stress, and maintain your motivation.

9. **Visualize Your Success:** Spend time visualizing your success and the positive outcomes of achieving your weight loss goals. Visualization can reinforce your determination and make your goals feel more attainable.

10. **Keep a Journal:** Consider keeping a journal to track your progress, thoughts, and feelings throughout your mindful eating journey. Reflecting on your experiences can offer insights and motivation.

As you continue your exploration of mindful eating and weight management, remember that motivation is a dynamic force that can ebb and flow. It's essential to nurture and maintain it along the way. Whether you find inspiration in your own progress, the stories of others, or the positive impact on your health, motivation will be your guiding light on this transformative path.

Now that you're armed with the truth about mindful eating, inspired by real-life success stories, and motivated to reach your weight loss goals, you're ready to continue your journey. Stay committed to your well-being, and keep these sources of motivation close to your heart as you move forward.

If you have any specific questions or need further guidance on your mindful eating journey, please don't hesitate to reach out. We're in this together, and your success is our shared goal.

Chapter 4: The Emotional Connection to Food

Welcome to Chapter 4, where we're about to embark on a deeply emotional journey. Get ready to explore the intricate and sometimes complex relationship between our emotions and the food we eat.

Emotions and Food: Uncovering the Intriguing Relationship

Emotions and food—two seemingly unrelated aspects of our lives that are often deeply intertwined. Have you ever found yourself reaching for a tub of ice cream after a tough day at work or craving your favorite comfort food when you're feeling down? If so, you're not alone.

In this chapter, we're going to unravel the fascinating connection between our emotions and our food choices. Let's dive right in.

Food as Comfort

For many of us, food serves as a source of comfort during challenging times. It's not just about satisfying physical hunger; it's about seeking solace in the flavors and textures that evoke feelings of warmth and security. Think about the homemade chicken soup your grandmother used to make when you were sick or the gooey macaroni and cheese that always put a smile on your face as a child.

Food can provide a sense of familiarity and nostalgia that soothes our emotions. It's like a warm hug in edible form. But here's where it gets tricky: relying solely on food for emotional comfort can lead to unhealthy eating patterns and weight gain.

Emotional Eating: A Double-Edged Sword

Emotional eating is a term you've probably heard before, and it describes the act of using food to cope with emotions, whether they're positive or negative. It's not inherently bad; we've all turned to food for comfort at some point in our lives. However, when emotional eating becomes a habitual response to every emotional twist and turn, it can lead to overeating and weight issues.

Mindful eating steps in as a valuable tool to address emotional eating. By practicing mindfulness, you'll become more attuned to your emotions and the triggers that lead to emotional eating. Instead of reaching for food automatically, you'll pause and ask yourself, "Am I truly hungry, or am I seeking comfort?"

The Power of Mindfulness

Mindfulness allows you to acknowledge your emotions without judgment. It teaches you to sit with your feelings, whether they're happiness, sadness, stress, or boredom, without using food as a crutch. Instead of suppressing emotions with calories, you'll develop healthier ways to cope.

Imagine this scenario: You've had a particularly challenging day at work, and your instinct is to grab a bag of chips and munch away your frustration. With mindfulness, you'll pause and take a moment to identify the emotions you're experiencing. You might realize that it's stress or anger driving your craving. Instead of eating, you could choose to practice deep breathing, take a short walk, or engage in a soothing activity like reading or listening to music. This shift from emotional eating to mindful coping is empowering.

Emotional Hunger vs. Physical Hunger

One of the key lessons in mindful eating is distinguishing between emotional hunger and physical hunger. They manifest differently:

- **Physical Hunger:** Physical hunger builds gradually and is typically accompanied by physical cues like a growling stomach, low energy, and an empty feeling. When you eat in response to physical hunger, you're nourishing your body's genuine needs.
- **Emotional Hunger:** Emotional hunger comes on suddenly and is often linked to specific emotions or situations. It's a craving for a particular food, such as chocolate or chips, and it's driven by the desire for emotional comfort rather than physical nourishment.

By learning to recognize the difference between these two types of hunger, you can make conscious choices about how to respond. Mindful eating encourages you to eat when you're physically hungry and address emotional needs through non-food means when necessary.

Breaking the Cycle of Emotional Eating

Breaking the cycle of emotional eating isn't easy, but it's entirely possible with mindfulness as your ally. Here are some strategies to help you overcome emotional eating:

1. **Keep a Food Diary:** Maintain a journal to track your eating patterns and the emotions associated with your meals and snacks. This can help you identify triggers and patterns.
2. **Practice Mindful Breathing:** When emotions threaten to overwhelm you, practice deep breathing exercises to center yourself and regain emotional balance.
3. **Seek Support:** Share your journey with a trusted friend, family member, or therapist who can provide emotional support and guidance.
4. **Mindful Distractions:** Develop a list of non-food activities that bring you joy and comfort. When emotional eating urges strike, engage in one of these activities instead.
5. **Slow Down and Savor:** When you do choose to eat, eat mindfully. Slow down, savor each bite, and fully experience the flavors and textures. This can help you become more attuned to physical hunger and fullness cues.

Remember, addressing emotional eating is a process, and it may take time and practice. Be patient with yourself, and approach it with self-compassion. As you continue your journey through the emotional landscape of eating, mindfulness will be your guide, helping you navigate the complexities of your emotions and food in a healthier, more balanced way.

Are you ready to dive deeper into this emotional connection to food and discover how mindfulness can transform your relationship with both? In the chapters ahead, we'll explore practical exercises and real-life stories to inspire and empower you on your path to mindful eating.

Recognizing Emotional Triggers

Emotional eating triggers can be subtle and elusive, often making us reach for food without conscious awareness. These triggers can be categorized into various emotional states and situations:

1. **Stress:** Stress is one of the most common triggers for emotional eating. When faced with stressors like work deadlines, relationship conflicts, or financial worries, many of us turn to food as a coping mechanism. Stress eating can temporarily provide comfort and distraction, but it doesn't address the root causes of stress.
2. **Sadness:** Feelings of sadness, loneliness, or grief can lead to emotional eating. Comfort foods, often high in sugar and fat, are sought to provide solace. These foods can temporarily elevate mood due to their impact on brain chemistry, but the relief is short-lived and followed by guilt.
3. **Boredom:** Boredom can be a powerful trigger for mindless eating. When there's a lack of engagement or stimulation, snacking becomes an activity to fill the void. This type of eating isn't driven by physical hunger but rather a desire for something to do.
4. **Anxiety:** Anxiety can lead to restlessness and a sense of unease, which some people attempt to soothe with food. The act of eating can create a temporary distraction from anxious thoughts, but it doesn't address the underlying anxiety.
5. **Celebration:** Surprisingly, positive emotions can also trigger emotional eating. Celebratory occasions, such as birthdays, promotions, or holidays, often involve indulgent foods. While there's nothing wrong with enjoying special treats, overindulging can lead to guilt and a sense of loss of control.
6. **Social Pressure:** Social situations can trigger emotional eating, especially when there's pressure to conform to social norms or expectations. For example, you might eat more than you want to at a

party to fit in or avoid drawing attention to yourself.

7. **Environmental Cues:** Sometimes, our environment can trigger eating without us even realizing it. The smell of freshly baked cookies, the sight of a vending machine, or the sound of a popcorn machine at the movies can prompt us to eat out of habit.

How Mindfulness Can Help

Mindfulness plays a pivotal role in recognizing and managing emotional eating triggers. Here's how:

1. **Increased Awareness:** Mindfulness involves being fully present in the moment. When you practice mindfulness, you become more aware of your emotions, thoughts, and physical sensations. This heightened awareness allows you to recognize emotional triggers as they arise.

2. **Mindful Pause:** Instead of reacting impulsively to emotions with food, mindfulness encourages you to take a mindful pause. When you feel an emotional trigger, pause and check in with yourself. Ask, "What am I feeling right now? Why do I want to eat?" This simple act of pausing can disrupt the automatic response of emotional eating.

3. **Non-Judgmental Observation:** Mindfulness invites non-judgmental observation of your emotions. Rather than labeling emotions as good or bad, you observe them with curiosity and compassion. This non-judgmental stance can reduce the shame and guilt often associated with emotional eating.

4. **Emotional Regulation:** Mindfulness equips you with tools to regulate your emotions without turning to food. Techniques like deep breathing, progressive muscle relaxation, and meditation can help you manage stress, anxiety, and other emotions in healthier ways.

5. **Mindful Eating:** Mindful eating practices can also be applied to emotional eating. Before reaching for food, ask yourself if you're physically hungry or if it's an emotional craving. If it's the latter, explore alternative ways to address the emotion, such as journaling,

talking to a friend, or engaging in a creative activity.

Mindful Reflection

As you continue your journey toward mindful eating, take a moment to reflect on your own emotional triggers. Consider the emotions or situations that tend to lead you to eat emotionally. Are there specific patterns you've noticed in your eating habits?

By recognizing these triggers, you're taking the first step toward managing emotional eating with mindfulness. Remember that it's a process, and it's okay to seek support and practice self-compassion along the way. In the following chapters, we'll delve deeper into practical exercises and strategies to help you navigate the complexities of emotional eating and build a healthier relationship with food.

As you embark on this exploration, know that you have the power to transform your relationship with food and emotions through mindfulness. You're not alone on this journey, and with each step, you're moving closer to a place of greater balance and well-being.

The Common Struggle: Emotional Eating

Before we dive into how mindfulness can be a game-changer, let's acknowledge that emotional eating is something most of us have experienced at one point or another. It's a natural response to our complex emotional lives. When we're stressed, sad, anxious, or even overly joyful, we may turn to food for comfort or distraction.

However, emotional eating often leads to a cycle of guilt and regret. We may consume food mindlessly, without truly savoring it, and afterward, we might feel worse than before. This cycle can have a significant impact on our physical and emotional well-being.

The Mindfulness Approach

Mindfulness, as you've learned, is about being fully present in the moment without judgment. This quality of presence can be a powerful antidote to emotional eating. Here's how:

1. **Awareness of Triggers:** Mindfulness helps us become aware of our emotional triggers. It encourages us to pause and examine what we're feeling when the urge to eat strikes. Are we truly hungry, or is there an underlying emotion at play?

2. **Recognizing the Urge:** When we practice mindfulness, we become skilled at recognizing the urge to eat in response to emotions. We notice the impulse as it arises, without immediately acting on it. This pause is crucial.

3. **Embracing Emotions:** Mindfulness doesn't judge our emotions as good or bad; it simply invites us to acknowledge them. Instead of suppressing or numbing our feelings with food, we learn to sit with them, understanding that emotions, like clouds, come and go.

4. **Alternative Coping Strategies:** Mindfulness equips us with alternative coping strategies for dealing with emotions. Instead of reaching for a bag of chips when stressed, we might engage in deep breathing, take a short walk, or practice meditation to calm the mind.

5. **Mindful Eating:** Even when we do choose to eat, mindfulness guides us in how we eat. We savor each bite, paying attention to the flavors, textures, and sensations. This mindful approach allows us to fully enjoy our food and recognize when we're satisfied.

Breaking the Cycle

Breaking the cycle of emotional eating with mindfulness involves a gradual shift in our relationship with emotions and food. It's a journey of self-discovery and self-compassion. Here are some practical steps to get you started:

1. **Pause and Identify:** When you feel the urge to eat in response to emotions, pause for a moment. Identify the emotion you're experiencing. Name it, if you can. Are you feeling stressed, anxious, sad, or bored?

2. **Breathe:** Take a few slow, deep breaths. This simple act can help calm your nervous system and create a mental space between the emotion and your response.

3. **Question the Urge:** Ask yourself, "Am I physically hungry right now?" This question helps you distinguish between emotional hunger and physical hunger. If you're not physically hungry, consider what other actions might soothe or address the emotion.

4. **Embrace the Emotion:** Instead of pushing the emotion away, allow yourself to feel it fully. Emotions are a natural part of the human experience. They won't harm you, and they won't last forever. Let them flow through you.

5. **Choose Mindful Coping:** Engage in a mindfulness practice that suits the situation. It could be as simple as taking a few mindful breaths or practicing a brief meditation. Experiment with various techniques to find what works best for you.

Your Mindful Journey

Remember, conquering emotional eating with mindfulness is not about perfection; it's about progress. Be patient with yourself as you explore these techniques. Over time, you'll develop greater self-awareness and resilience in the face of emotional triggers.

As you continue your journey through the complexities of emotional eating, keep in mind that mindfulness is your ally. It empowers you to make conscious choices, nurture self-compassion, and build a healthier relationship with both your emotions and food.

So, are you ready to embrace mindfulness as a tool to conquer emotional eating? The path ahead may have its challenges, but it also holds the promise of greater self-awareness, inner strength, and freedom from the cycle of emotional eating. Your journey is unique, and you have the capacity to transform your relationship with food and emotions for the better.

Strategies to Handle Emotional Eating with Grace and Self-Compassion

Emotional eating is a complex and often deeply ingrained habit. It's not something that can be overcome overnight, but with mindfulness, self-compassion, and the right strategies, you can navigate this challenge with grace and resilience.

1. Mindful Awareness: The first step in managing emotional eating is to develop mindful awareness. This involves paying close attention to your thoughts, emotions, and physical sensations when the urge to eat in response to emotions arises. When you become aware of these triggers, you gain the power to respond rather than react.

2. Journaling: Keeping a journal can be a powerful tool for understanding your emotional eating patterns. When you feel the urge to eat emotionally, take a moment to write down what you're feeling, what triggered the emotion, and how you responded. Over time, patterns may emerge that shed light on your emotional eating habits.

3. Emotional Regulation Techniques: To break free from emotional eating, it's essential to have alternative strategies for managing your emotions. Experiment with techniques such as deep breathing exercises, progressive muscle relaxation, or mindfulness meditation. These practices can help you regulate your emotions without turning to food.

4. Self-Compassion: Self-compassion is a key component of handling emotional eating gracefully. Treat yourself with the same kindness and understanding you would offer to a dear friend facing a similar challenge. Instead of berating yourself for emotional eating episodes, approach them with self-compassion and a commitment to learning and growth.

5. Seek Support: You don't have to go through this journey alone. Reach out to a therapist, counselor, or support group that specializes in emotional eating and mindful approaches to eating. Sharing your experiences and receiving guidance from others can be incredibly empowering.

6. Mindful Coping Strategies: Develop a toolkit of mindful coping strategies that resonate with you. These strategies should be readily available when you're faced with emotional triggers. Some people find solace in art, journaling, listening to music, or going for a walk. Experiment with various activities to discover what helps you manage emotions effectively.

7. Slow and Steady: Remember that breaking the cycle of emotional eating is a gradual process. Be patient with yourself, and celebrate small victories along the way. Each time you respond to emotional triggers with mindfulness and self-compassion, you're making progress.

Personal Stories: We're All in This Together

It's reassuring to know that you're not alone in your journey to conquer emotional eating. Many individuals have faced and overcome this challenge, and their personal stories can offer inspiration, guidance, and a sense of solidarity.

Emma's Story: Emma, a 35-year-old marketing executive, struggled with stress-related emotional eating for years. She would often reach for sugary snacks during high-pressure workdays. Through mindfulness practices and therapy, Emma learned to recognize her stress triggers and respond with self-compassion. She now takes short mindful breaks during the workday, practices deep breathing, and engages in regular yoga sessions. Emma's story reminds us that with mindfulness and self-care, it's possible to break free from the grip of emotional eating.

Tom's Journey: Tom, a 42-year-old teacher, used food as a way to cope with feelings of loneliness and boredom. He realized that emotional eating was holding him back from living a healthier life. With the support of a mindful eating group, Tom learned to distinguish between physical hunger and emotional cravings. He also discovered the joy of cooking and started preparing balanced meals that nourished both his body and soul. Tom's story illustrates that connecting with a supportive community can be a game-changer on the path to mindful eating.

Sara's Transformation: Sara, a 29-year-old graphic designer, found herself turning to food for comfort when dealing with anxiety and self-doubt. Mindfulness meditation became a cornerstone of her journey. It helped her cultivate self-awareness and self-compassion. Sara also adopted a practice of mindful eating, savoring each bite and tuning in to her body's hunger and fullness cues. With time, she developed a healthier relationship with food and a newfound sense of inner peace. Sara's story demonstrates the transformative potential of mindfulness in overcoming emotional eating.

These personal stories highlight the diversity of experiences and paths toward mindful eating. They serve as a reminder that emotional eating is a shared challenge, and there are strategies and support systems available to help you navigate it.

As you continue on your journey to conquer emotional eating with grace and self-compassion, draw inspiration from these stories. Embrace the fact that you're not alone, and that like Emma, Tom, and Sara, you too can find your unique path to mindful eating.

In the chapters ahead, we'll delve deeper into practical exercises and insights to empower you on your journey toward a healthier relationship with food and emotions.

Chapter 5: Mindful Eating in a Fast-Paced World

Welcome to Chapter 5, where we'll explore the art of mindful eating in the midst of our fast-paced modern world. You might be thinking, "Is it even possible to eat mindfully when life moves at such a rapid pace?" The answer is a resounding yes. In this chapter, we'll tackle the modern-day challenges of eating mindfully head-on.

The Modern-Day Challenges of Eating Mindfully

Our lives have become increasingly fast-paced, and it often feels like we're constantly juggling multiple tasks and responsibilities. In the midst of this whirlwind, finding time for mindful eating can indeed seem like a daunting task. However, it's essential to understand that the very pace of our lives makes mindfulness all the more crucial.

Let's explore some of the common challenges and misconceptions associated with eating mindfully in a fast-paced world:

1. The Myth of Multitasking: Many of us believe that multitasking is the key to efficiency. We eat while working, watching TV, or scrolling through our phones. While it may seem productive, multitasking during meals often leads to mindless eating. We lose touch with the sensory experience of eating, and our body's hunger and fullness cues go unnoticed.

2. Time Constraints: Busy schedules can create the illusion that we don't have time to eat mindfully. Rushed mornings, back-to-back meetings, and tight deadlines may make it challenging to sit down for a leisurely meal. As a result, we resort to quick, on-the-go options that don't promote mindful eating.

3. External Distractions: Our environment is filled with distractions that pull our attention away from our plates. Whether it's the noise of a bustling cafe, the TV blaring in the background, or the notifications on our devices, these external distractions hinder our ability to fully engage with our meals.

4. Social Pressure: Social occasions and group meals can also pose challenges to mindful eating. The desire to fit in or the fear of appearing different may lead us to abandon our mindful eating practices in favor of social norms.

5. Instant Gratification Culture: We live in a world where speed and convenience are highly valued. Fast food, instant meals, and grab-and-go snacks are readily available, but they often lack the nourishment and satisfaction that come from mindful eating.

Tackling the Challenges Head-On

The good news is that while these challenges are real, they are not insurmountable. Mindful eating can be woven into the fabric of our fast-paced lives with some intentional shifts in perspective and habits. Here's how:

1. Prioritize Mindful Meals: Start by recognizing the importance of mindful eating in your overall well-being. Make it a priority to set aside time for at least one mindful meal each day. Even if it's just a few minutes, it can make a significant difference.

2. Create Mindful Spaces: Whenever possible, choose a calm and quiet environment for your meals. Turn off distractions like the TV and put away your devices. Create a sacred space for eating, even if it's just a corner of your kitchen table.

3. Single-Tasking: Embrace the practice of single-tasking during meals. When you eat, eat. Focus solely on the act of nourishing yourself. Avoid working, scrolling, or watching TV while you dine.

4. Mindful Snacking: If you find it challenging to allocate time for full meals, consider incorporating mindfulness into your snacking habits. Choose nutritious snacks and take a moment to savor their flavors and textures.

5. Mindful on the Go: For those moments when eating on the go is inevitable, bring mindfulness with you. Pause before taking your first bite, take a few deep breaths, and express gratitude for your meal. Even in a rush, you can infuse a touch of mindfulness into your eating.

6. Social Mindfulness: When dining with others, communicate your commitment to mindful eating. Encourage your friends and family to join you in savoring the meal. Sharing the practice can make it more enjoyable and less isolating.

7. Embrace Imperfection: Finally, remember that mindful eating is not about perfection. It's about intention and awareness. There will be days when the pace of life feels overwhelming, and that's okay. Approach mindful eating with a gentle and forgiving spirit.

Mindfulness in Motion

In a fast-paced world, the practice of mindful eating becomes a form of mindfulness in motion. It's a way of grounding yourself in the present moment, even when life seems to be racing by. By recognizing and addressing the challenges of eating mindfully in a fast-paced world, you can reclaim a sense of balance and nourishment in your daily life.

As you continue your journey through this chapter, consider how you can apply these principles to your own life. Remember that mindful eating is not an all-or-nothing endeavor. Every moment of mindfulness counts, and each step brings you closer to a healthier and more fulfilling relationship with food.

Practical Tips for Bringing Mindfulness into Your Hectic Life

1. **The Power of Pause:** Begin your day with a mindful pause. Instead of jumping out of bed and rushing into your daily routine, take a few moments to lie still, breathe deeply, and set an intention for the day ahead. This simple practice can help you start your day with greater presence and clarity.

2. **Mindful Morning Routine:** Turn your morning routine into a mindfulness ritual. Whether it's showering, brushing your teeth, or making coffee, approach each task with full attention. Notice the sensations, smells, and sounds involved in these everyday activities.

3. **Mindful Commuting:** If your schedule involves a daily commute, use this time as an opportunity for mindfulness. Instead of getting lost in thoughts or distractions, focus on your breath or the sights and

sounds around you. This can transform a mundane commute into a mindful journey.

4. **Mindful Eating Moments:** Even if you can't set aside extended periods for mindful meals, you can infuse moments of mindfulness into your eating. Before taking a bite, pause for a breath and express gratitude for your food. Chew slowly, savoring each bite, and pay attention to the flavors and textures.

5. **Micro-Mindfulness:** Incorporate micro-mindfulness throughout your day. Take short breaks to tune into your breath, check in with your body, or simply appreciate a moment of stillness. These brief pauses can reset your mind and reduce stress.

6. **Mindful Technology Use:** Given our reliance on technology, aim to use it mindfully. Set boundaries for screen time and notifications, and take regular tech breaks to recenter yourself. This can improve your focus and reduce digital distractions.

7. **Mindful Transitions:** Mindfulness can be integrated into transitions between tasks or activities. Before moving from one task to another, take a moment to breathe deeply and reset your focus. This practice can enhance your efficiency and reduce mental clutter.

8. **Mindful Evening Reflection:** As your day winds down, engage in a mindful reflection. Take a few minutes to review your day, acknowledging both the challenges and the moments of gratitude. This practice can promote a sense of closure and relaxation.

9. **Mindful Sleep:** Prioritize mindful sleep by creating a calming bedtime routine. Dim the lights, disconnect from screens, and engage in relaxation techniques like gentle stretching or meditation to prepare your mind and body for restful sleep.

10. **Mindful Mini-Retreats:** Occasionally, set aside small pockets of time for mini-retreats. Even 10-15 minutes of mindfulness meditation or deep breathing can provide a refreshing break and enhance your overall well-being.

Customize Your Mindfulness Routine

Remember that mindfulness is highly adaptable and can be tailored to your unique schedule and preferences. Experiment with different practices to discover what resonates with you. The key is to approach each moment with intention and presence, regardless of how brief it may be.

By infusing your hectic schedule with mindfulness, you can cultivate a sense of balance, reduce stress, and enhance your overall quality of life. You don't need to find extra hours in the day to be mindful; you can transform everyday moments into opportunities for greater awareness and well-being.

As you navigate the challenges of your busy life, keep these practical tips in mind and be open to the transformative power of mindfulness in even the most fast-paced moments.

Mindful Eating: Your Stress Reduction Tool

Stress has become an all-too-common companion in our fast-paced lives. Whether it's work-related pressures, personal challenges, or the demands of daily living, stress can take a toll on both our mental and physical health. The good news is that mindful eating can serve as a valuable tool for stress reduction.

1. Mindful Presence: When you engage in mindful eating, you bring your full attention to the present moment. This means letting go of worries about the past or future and immersing yourself in the sensory experience of eating. By doing so, you create a mental refuge from the stressors of life.

2. Stress Hormone Regulation: Chronic stress can lead to the overproduction of stress hormones like cortisol. Mindful eating promotes relaxation and activates the body's relaxation response, counteracting the negative effects of stress hormones. This can help reduce anxiety and promote a sense of calm.

3. Reduced Emotional Eating: Mindful eating helps you become more aware of your emotional triggers for eating. Instead of turning to food as a coping mechanism for stress, you can respond to emotional challenges in a healthier way. This reduces the likelihood of emotional overeating.

4. Improved Digestion: Stress can disrupt digestion and lead to issues like indigestion or irritable bowel syndrome. Mindful eating encourages a state of relaxation, which supports optimal digestion and absorption of nutrients.

5. Enhanced Satisfaction: Rushed and distracted eating often leaves us feeling unsatisfied, leading to cravings and overeating. Mindful eating allows you to fully savor each bite, enhancing the satisfaction you derive from your meals. This can reduce the urge to snack on unhealthy foods in response to stress.

Mindful Eating as a Stress Ritual

To harness the stress-reducing power of mindful eating, consider adopting it as a regular ritual in your life:

1. Start Small: Begin with one meal or snack per day that you can commit to eating mindfully. It could be your morning coffee, a piece of fruit, or your lunch break. As you become more comfortable with the practice, you can expand it to other meals.

2. Create a Calm Environment: Choose a quiet, clutter-free space for your mindful meals. Turn off distractions like the TV or your phone, and create an atmosphere that promotes relaxation.

3. Deep Breathing: Begin your mindful meal with a few deep breaths to center yourself. This can help you transition from a state of stress to one of calm focus.

4. Engage the Senses: As you eat, engage all your senses. Notice the colors, textures, and aromas of your food. Pay attention to the sounds as you chew and the flavors that unfold on your palate.

5. Slow Down: Eat slowly and deliberately. Take small bites and chew thoroughly. Put your utensils down between bites to fully savor each morsel.

6. Be Present: Bring your full attention to the experience of eating. If your mind starts to wander, gently guide it back to the present moment. Avoid distractions and judgments.

7. Express Gratitude: Before and after your meal, take a moment to express gratitude for the food and the opportunity to nourish yourself. This practice can foster a positive mindset and reduce stress.

8. Practice Regularly: Consistency is key. The more you incorporate mindful eating into your routine, the more effective it becomes as a stress-reduction tool.

By making mindful eating a part of your life, you can not only improve your relationship with food but also build resilience against the daily stressors that come your way. It's a simple yet powerful practice that can have a profound impact on your overall well-being.

As you explore the stress-reducing benefits of mindful eating, remember that it's a journey of self-discovery and self-care. Embrace it with patience and compassion, and you'll find that it becomes an essential tool in your stress management toolkit.

Eating Mindfully at Work or On the Go

Many of us spend a significant portion of our day at work or are constantly on the move, making it seem challenging to incorporate mindfulness into our eating habits. However, with a bit of intention and creativity, you can practice mindful eating even in these busy settings.

1. Mindful Work Lunch: If you're eating at your desk or in a work environment, set the stage for mindful eating by creating a calm workspace. Turn off notifications on your devices, and if possible, step away from your desk to eat in a quiet spot. Use this time as an opportunity to take a break from work-related stressors.

2. Pack Mindful Snacks: For those on the go, consider packing mindful snacks like a small container of nuts, a piece of fruit, or a yogurt cup. These portable options allow you to enjoy a nutritious snack mindfully without feeling rushed.

3. Slow Down: Whether you're at work or out and about, remind yourself to slow down. Avoid the temptation to rush through your meal or snack. Take deliberate bites, chew slowly, and savor the flavors. This not only promotes mindfulness but also helps with digestion and satisfaction.

4. Mindful Sips: If you're sipping on a beverage, whether it's a morning coffee or a mid-afternoon tea, use this moment to practice mindfulness. Feel the warmth of the cup in your hands, inhale the aroma, and take small, deliberate sips, fully experiencing the taste and texture.

5. Mindful Breaks: Instead of using your breaks to check emails or scroll through social media, consider using them for mindfulness breaks. Find a quiet space, close your eyes, and take a few minutes to focus on your breath or perform a quick body scan to release tension.

Quick Mindfulness Exercises for Busy Bees

In addition to mindful eating, incorporating quick mindfulness exercises into your daily routine can help you stay grounded and reduce stress, even during the busiest of days:

1. Three-Minute Breathing: Find a quiet spot, close your eyes, and take three minutes to focus solely on your breath. Inhale deeply through your nose for a count of four, hold for a count of four, and exhale for a count of four. Repeat this cycle, allowing your breath to anchor you in the present moment.

2. Five Senses Check-In: Take a moment to engage your five senses. What can you see, hear, smell, taste, and touch in your current environment? This exercise can help you shift your awareness away from racing thoughts and into the sensory experience of the present.

3. Mini-Mindful Walk: If you have a short break, go for a mini-mindful walk. Focus on the sensation of your feet hitting the ground, the rhythm of your steps, and the sights and sounds around you. It's a simple way to recharge and reconnect with the world outside of work.

4. Desk Mindfulness: Even at your desk, you can practice mindfulness. Take a minute to close your eyes and take three deep breaths. With each breath, let go of any tension or stress you may be holding onto.

5. Mindful Snacking: If you have a snack at hand, use it as an opportunity for a brief mindfulness exercise. Engage your senses by exploring the colors, textures, and flavors of your snack. Eat slowly and savor each bite.

By incorporating these tips and quick mindfulness exercises into your workday or on-the-go routine, you can maintain a sense of balance, reduce stress, and enhance your overall well-being. Remember that mindfulness doesn't always require extended periods of time; even brief moments of presence can make a significant difference in your day.

Chapter 6: Mindful Eating for Improved Digestion

Welcome to Chapter 6, where we delve into the intriguing connection between mindful eating and your digestive system's well-being. If you've ever wondered how mindfulness can benefit your grumbly tummy and promote better digestion, you're in the right place. Let's explore the ways in which mindful eating can work wonders for your digestive health.

The Mind-Gut Connection

Before we dive into the specifics of mindful eating and digestion, it's essential to understand the fascinating mind-gut connection. Your brain and your digestive system are in constant communication, and this bidirectional link plays a pivotal role in your overall well-being.

Have you ever experienced a "gut feeling" or noticed that stress can lead to digestive discomfort? These experiences highlight the intricate connection between your thoughts, emotions, and your gut. Stress, anxiety, and negative emotions can trigger digestive issues, while a relaxed state of mind can promote optimal digestion.

How Mindful Eating Supports Digestion

Mindful eating aligns perfectly with the mind-gut connection, fostering an environment that supports healthy digestion. Here's how it works:

1. Stress Reduction: Mindful eating encourages a state of relaxation during meals. When you're calm and present, your body is in a better position to digest food effectively. By reducing stress and anxiety during mealtime, you can prevent common digestive complaints like indigestion and bloating.

2. Improved Chewing: Mindful eaters tend to chew their food more thoroughly. This simple act of chewing each bite thoroughly breaks down food into smaller, more manageable pieces. This not only aids in digestion but also ensures that your stomach doesn't have to work as hard.

3. Enhanced Nutrient Absorption: When you eat mindfully, you become more attuned to the flavors, textures, and smells of your food. This sensory awareness extends to your body's ability to detect and absorb nutrients. By savoring the experience of eating, you can improve nutrient absorption and overall nourishment.

4. Portion Control: Mindful eating promotes awareness of hunger and fullness cues. This means you're less likely to overeat, which can put undue stress on your digestive system. Eating until you're satisfied, not stuffed, is a key principle of mindful eating that supports optimal digestion.

5. Reduced Binge Eating: For those who struggle with binge eating or emotional overeating, mindful eating offers a path to breaking these unhealthy patterns. By addressing the emotional component of eating, you can reduce the likelihood of overloading your digestive system with excess food.

Mindful Eating Practices for Digestive Health

Now that you understand how mindful eating can benefit your digestion let's explore some specific practices that can promote a happier, healthier gut:

1. Mindful Meal Preparation: Approach meal preparation with mindfulness. Take your time selecting ingredients, notice their colors and textures, and savor the process of cooking. This mindful approach extends the benefits of mindfulness to your digestive experience.

2. Mindful Dining Environment: Create a peaceful dining environment that supports digestion. Avoid eating in front of the TV or computer. Instead, dine in a calm, clutter-free space with minimal distractions.

3. Breath Awareness: Before you start eating, take a few deep breaths to center yourself. This signals to your body that it's time to relax and digest. Focusing on your breath can be particularly beneficial during stressful or rushed meals.

4. Chew Thoroughly: Make a conscious effort to chew each bite thoroughly. Put down your utensils between bites to slow down the pace of your meal. Chewing well not only supports digestion but also enhances your enjoyment of food.

5. Savor the Flavors: Pay attention to the flavors and textures of your food as you eat. Notice how each bite evolves in your mouth. Engaging your senses can enhance the digestive process.

6. Mindful Eating Journal: Consider keeping a mindful eating journal to track your meals and your digestive experiences. Note any patterns or triggers that affect your digestion. This self-awareness can help you make informed choices.

7. Post-Meal Reflection: After finishing your meal, take a moment to reflect on how you feel. Are you comfortably satisfied? Do you notice any signs of discomfort? This reflection can inform your future eating choices.

By incorporating these mindful eating practices into your daily life, you can nurture a positive relationship between your mind and your digestive system. Improved digestion leads to greater comfort, better nutrient absorption, and overall well-being.

As we journey through this chapter, keep in mind that mindful eating is a valuable tool for promoting digestive health. Embrace these practices with an open heart and an open mind, and you'll find that your digestive system can become your ally in your quest for overall wellness.

Savoring Each Bite

Picture this: you're sitting down to a meal, and instead of mindlessly rushing through it, you take a deep breath and consciously engage with your food. You notice the colors, textures, and aromas on your plate. You pick up your fork or spoon deliberately and take your time to savor each bite.

This is the essence of mindful eating—a practice that prioritizes the quality of your eating experience over speed and mindlessness. It's an antidote to the rushed meals that can lead to a host of digestive issues, including indigestion, bloating, and discomfort.

The Mindful Eating Digestive Rescue

Here's how mindful eating comes to the rescue when it comes to your digestive health:

1. Stress Reduction: Rushed meals often go hand in hand with stress and anxiety. When you're in a hurry, your body is in a heightened state of stress, which can disrupt the digestive process. Mindful eating promotes relaxation, helping to ease the stress response and create a harmonious environment for digestion.

2. Better Chewing: Mindful eaters tend to chew their food more thoroughly. This is essential for digestion because the digestive process begins in your mouth. When you chew your food well, you break it down into smaller, more digestible particles, making it easier for your stomach and intestines to do their job.

3. Improved Nutrient Absorption: By paying close attention to the flavors and textures of your food, you become more aware of the entire eating experience. This heightened awareness extends to your body's ability to detect and absorb nutrients. When you're fully present, you're more likely to absorb the maximum nutritional benefit from your meal.

4. Portion Control: Rushed eating often leads to overeating, which can place unnecessary stress on your digestive system. Mindful eating encourages you to listen to your body's hunger and fullness cues, helping you eat until you're satisfied, not stuffed.

5. Reduced Binge Eating: For individuals who struggle with binge eating or emotional overeating, mindful eating offers a way out of these patterns. By acknowledging and addressing the emotional aspect of eating, you can prevent the discomfort and distress that often follow overindulgence.

A Digestive Health Revolution

As you embark on your mindful eating journey, you'll likely notice a significant shift in your digestive health. The discomfort and bloating that once plagued your post-meal experiences can become a thing of the past. Instead, you'll find yourself embracing a newfound sense of digestive ease and comfort.

Imagine saying goodbye to indigestion and hello to a digestive system that operates smoothly and efficiently. Picture meals that leave you feeling satisfied, not overstuffed, and a sense of well-being that accompanies every bite. This is the digestive health revolution that mindful eating can usher into your life.

Your Digestive Journey

As we navigate this chapter together, keep in mind that mindful eating is not a quick fix but a journey—a journey that invites you to explore the profound connection between your mind and your digestive system. It's a journey of self-discovery and self-care, where you learn to treat each meal as a precious opportunity to nurture your body and soul.

So, as you continue on this path of mindful eating, remember that it's a rescue mission—one that liberates you from the stress of rushed meals and digestive discomfort. Embrace it with open arms, and you'll find that your digestive system becomes your ally in the quest for overall wellness.

The Five Senses Feast:

This practice involves engaging all five of your senses to fully experience your meal. Begin by taking a moment to observe your food using your sense of sight. Notice the colors, shapes, and presentation of your meal. Then, inhale deeply to engage your sense of smell, taking in the aromas wafting from your plate. As you take your first bite, focus on the textures and flavors, savoring each mouthful. Listen to the sounds as you chew and swallow. This practice not only enhances your sensory experience but also promotes mindful eating.

The Mindful Bite:

The mindful bite is a simple yet powerful practice. Before taking a bite, pause for a moment and bring your full attention to the food in front of you. Observe it closely, noticing the details and textures. As you take your first bite, chew slowly and deliberately. Pay attention to the sensations in your mouth as the flavors unfold. Try to identify the different tastes and textures in each bite. This practice encourages you to savor each morsel and promotes thorough chewing, which aids digestion.

The Gratitude Ritual:

Before and after your meal, take a moment to express gratitude. Begin by acknowledging the effort that went into preparing your meal, whether by yourself or others. As you eat, feel thankful for the nourishment that the food provides. This practice helps shift your focus to a positive mindset, reducing stress and creating a harmonious environment for digestion.

The Mindful Pause:

The mindful pause is a practice that you can incorporate throughout your meal. It involves setting down your utensils between bites and taking a moment to check in with yourself. Pause to assess your hunger and fullness levels. Are you still genuinely hungry, or are you satisfied? This practice prevents overeating and helps you stay attuned to your body's signals.

The Breath of Ease:

During your meal, periodically pause to take a few deep breaths. This simple act can signal to your body that it's time to relax and focus on digestion. Inhale deeply through your nose, hold for a moment, and exhale slowly through your mouth. As you breathe, let go of any tension or stress. This practice promotes a relaxed state of mind and body, enhancing the digestive process.

The Post-Meal Reflection:

After finishing your meal, take a moment to reflect on how you feel. Are you comfortably satisfied, or do you feel overly full? Notice any sensations in your stomach and digestive tract. This post-meal reflection allows you to assess your eating habits and make adjustments as needed. It's a valuable tool for maintaining digestive comfort.

The Mindful Beverage Break:

If you're enjoying a beverage with your meal, whether it's water, tea, or another beverage of your choice, use it as an opportunity for mindfulness. Pay attention to the temperature and taste of your drink. Take deliberate sips, savoring each one. This practice complements your meal, enhancing your overall dining experience.

By incorporating these mindful practices into your meals, you can supercharge your digestion and foster a deeper connection with the food you eat. These practices not only promote digestive health but also enrich your culinary journey, making each meal a source of joy and nourishment. So, dive in, experiment with these practices, and discover how mindful eating can truly transform your digestive well-being.

Better Food Choices: The Foundation of Digestive Health

When it comes to digestive well-being, the quality and composition of your meals play a pivotal role. Making better food choices is not about restrictive diets or deprivation; it's about choosing foods that support your overall health and digestion. Here are some key principles to consider:

1. Whole, Unprocessed Foods: Opt for whole, unprocessed foods whenever possible. These foods are rich in nutrients, fiber, and natural goodness. Fruits, vegetables, whole grains, lean proteins, and healthy fats should be staples on your plate.

2. Mindful Portion Sizes: Pay attention to portion sizes. Mindful eating encourages you to eat until you're satisfied, not stuffed. This practice not only supports digestion but also helps with weight management.

3. Balanced Meals: Aim for balanced meals that include a variety of nutrients. A well-balanced plate typically consists of a protein source, a generous portion of colorful vegetables, a serving of whole grains, and healthy fats. This combination provides essential nutrients and promotes digestive comfort.

4. Hydration: Proper hydration is essential for digestion. Water helps break down food in your stomach and facilitates the movement of food through your digestive tract. Ensure you're drinking enough water throughout the day to support optimal digestion.

5. Mindful Snacking: If you enjoy snacks between meals, choose mindful options. Opt for snacks that provide sustained energy and nourishment, such as a handful of nuts, a piece of fruit, or yogurt. Avoid highly processed and sugary snacks that can disrupt digestion.

6. Dietary Fiber: Incorporate fiber-rich foods into your diet. Fiber supports healthy digestion by promoting regular bowel movements and preventing constipation. Whole grains, legumes, fruits, and vegetables are excellent sources of dietary fiber.

7. Probiotics: Consider including foods rich in probiotics, such as yogurt, kefir, sauerkraut, and kimchi. Probiotics promote a healthy balance of gut bacteria, which is essential for digestive health.

Real-Life Digestive Transformations

As we explore these principles of mindful food choices, we'll continue to be inspired by real-life stories of individuals who have experienced remarkable transformations in their digestion through mindfulness.

Imagine hearing the journey of someone who, like you, struggled with digestive discomfort, bloating, or indigestion. They found relief and improved digestive health by embracing mindful eating practices and making conscious food choices. These stories serve as a source of motivation and encouragement on your own digestive wellness journey.

So, let's delve into the world of mindful food choices and real-life digestive transformations. Together, we'll uncover the power of mindful eating not only as a tool for improved digestion but also as a pathway to overall health and well-being.

Real-Life Transformation 1: Sarah's Journey to Digestive Freedom

Meet Sarah, a busy professional who, like many of us, struggled with digestive discomfort for years. Her days were often marked by bloating, gas, and irregular bowel movements, making her work and social life challenging. She tried various diets and over-the-counter remedies, but nothing provided lasting relief.

Sarah's turning point came when she discovered mindful eating. Through the practice of mindfulness, she learned to approach her meals with a sense of calm and presence. She began to pay close attention to the way her body responded to different foods, identifying triggers for her digestive issues.

By making mindful food choices and savoring each bite, Sarah found that she could prevent overeating and reduce the discomfort associated with her meals. She also noticed a correlation between stress and her digestive symptoms, which prompted her to incorporate stress-reduction techniques into her daily routine.

Over time, Sarah's digestion improved significantly. Her symptoms of bloating and gas became less frequent, and she enjoyed a newfound sense of digestive freedom. Through mindfulness, she not only transformed her relationship with food but also reclaimed her vitality and well-being.

Real-Life Transformation 2: Mark's Journey to Gut Health

Mark had been dealing with acid reflux and heartburn for years. These uncomfortable symptoms often left him sleepless and irritable. He relied on antacids and prescription medications to manage his condition, but the relief was temporary and came with side effects.

Mark decided to explore alternative approaches to address his digestive issues, and that's when he stumbled upon mindful eating. He began to practice eating with full awareness, taking time to chew each bite thoroughly and paying attention to the sensations in his stomach.

As he embraced mindful eating, Mark noticed that he was naturally making better food choices. He gravitated toward foods that were less likely to trigger his acid reflux. He also realized that eating mindfully helped him eat smaller, more manageable portions, reducing the pressure on his digestive system.

Over time, Mark's symptoms of acid reflux and heartburn diminished. He gradually reduced his reliance on medications, and his sleep improved significantly. Mark's journey to gut health was a testament to the transformative power of mindful eating in managing digestive conditions.

Real-Life Transformation 3: Emma's Path to Digestive Harmony

Emma had struggled with chronic constipation for as long as she could remember. She tried numerous remedies, from laxatives to dietary supplements, but her condition remained a constant source of discomfort and frustration.

Emma's journey toward digestive harmony began when she started practicing mindful eating. Through mindfulness, she became attuned to the signals of hunger and fullness in her body. She also learned to appreciate the importance of dietary fiber and hydration in supporting regular bowel movements.

By making mindful food choices and incorporating fiber-rich foods into her diet, Emma experienced a remarkable transformation. Her constipation gradually improved, and she no longer relied on medications or supplements. Emma's digestive system began to function more efficiently, and she felt a renewed sense of well-being.

These real-life digestive transformations highlight the potential of mindful eating as a powerful tool for improving digestive health. Whether it's overcoming bloating, managing acid reflux, or alleviating chronic constipation, mindfulness can lead to profound changes in how we experience and nourish our bodies. As you embark on your own mindful eating journey, let these stories inspire you, knowing that positive changes in your digestive health are well within reach.

Chapter 7: Mindful Eating and Food Choices

Welcome to Chapter 7, where we dive into the heart of mindful eating—how it guides the choices you make when it comes to what's on your plate. While mindful eating encompasses how you eat, it's equally about what you eat. In this chapter, we'll explore how mindfulness in action shapes our food choices and how this can transform your relationship with food and your overall well-being.

Mindfulness in Action: How It Guides Our Food Choices

Mindfulness extends its gentle influence beyond the act of eating itself; it plays a pivotal role in the very foods you select to nourish your body. Here's how mindfulness in action guides your food choices:

1. Heightened Awareness: Through mindfulness, you become more attuned to your body's signals, including hunger and fullness cues. This heightened awareness allows you to make food choices based on your body's true needs rather than emotional or impulsive desires. You'll find yourself selecting foods that genuinely satisfy and nourish you.

2. Sensory Engagement: Mindful eaters engage their senses fully when it comes to food. This means you savor the flavors, textures, and aromas of your meals. It's not just about mindlessly consuming calories; it's about relishing the sensory experience of eating. You'll naturally gravitate toward foods that provide both pleasure and sustenance.

3. The Mindful Pause: Before making a food choice, you're more likely to take a mindful pause. You'll consider your options and reflect on what your body truly craves at that moment. This prevents impulsive or habitual eating patterns and empowers you to make conscious decisions that align with your well-being.

4. Emotional Awareness: Mindful eating also involves recognizing the emotional component of food choices. You'll become aware of how emotions, such as stress, boredom, or joy, influence your cravings and eating habits. With this awareness, you can choose foods that address emotional needs without resorting to mindless or unhealthy eating.

5. Nutrient Value: Mindful eaters tend to prioritize nutrient-rich foods that support overall health. You'll naturally opt for foods that provide essential vitamins, minerals, fiber, and other nutrients. This ensures that your body receives the nourishment it needs to thrive.

6. Mindful Meal Planning: Planning your meals mindfully becomes a regular practice. You'll consider a balanced mix of foods that provide sustained energy and satiety. Mindful meal planning helps you avoid last-minute, less nutritious choices.

7. Gratitude and Respect: Mindful eating fosters a sense of gratitude for the food you choose. You develop a deep respect for the sources of your nourishment, whether it's the earth, farmers, or those who prepare your meals. This gratitude extends to making choices that honor your health and the environment.

The Mindful Eating Plate

Imagine creating your own mindful eating plate—a plate that reflects your commitment to nourishing your body and soul. It's a plate filled with colorful vegetables, whole grains, lean proteins, and healthy fats. Each meal becomes an opportunity to express gratitude and care for yourself through the foods you choose.

In this chapter, we'll explore practical tips and strategies for incorporating mindfulness into your food choices. You'll discover that mindful eating isn't about restriction but about making choices that align with your values and well-being.

So, as we journey through this chapter, remember that mindfulness in action guides not only how you eat but also what you eat. By embracing this holistic approach to food, you'll nourish your body, mind, and spirit in ways that promote lasting health and happiness.

The Power of Nutritious, Whole Foods

Nutritious, whole foods form the cornerstone of mindful eating. These foods, in their natural and unprocessed state, are packed with essential nutrients, vitamins, minerals, and dietary fiber. Let's take a closer look at their benefits:

1. Nutrient Density: Whole foods are nutrient-dense, meaning they provide a high concentration of essential nutrients relative to their calorie content. This ensures that your body receives the vital vitamins and minerals it needs for optimal function.

2. Sustained Energy: Whole foods are excellent sources of complex carbohydrates, which provide sustained energy. Unlike refined carbohydrates, which can lead to energy crashes, whole grains and starchy vegetables release energy slowly, keeping you feeling energized throughout the day.

3. Dietary Fiber: Fiber is abundant in whole foods like fruits, vegetables, legumes, and whole grains. Fiber supports digestive health by promoting regular bowel movements, preventing constipation, and fostering a healthy gut microbiome.

4. Satiety and Weight Management: Whole foods are often more filling and satisfying than processed alternatives. They help regulate hunger and fullness cues, making it easier to maintain a healthy weight and avoid overeating.

5. Disease Prevention: A diet rich in whole foods is associated with a lower risk of chronic diseases such as heart disease, diabetes, and certain types of cancer. The antioxidants and phytochemicals found in fruits and vegetables provide protection against oxidative stress and inflammation.

6. Improved Digestion: Whole foods, particularly those high in fiber, support digestive health. They aid in the efficient movement of food through the digestive tract and prevent issues like indigestion and bloating.

7. Mindful Eating: Whole foods are ideally suited for mindful eating practices. Their vibrant colors, textures, and flavors engage your senses, enhancing the mindful eating experience. You savor each bite, appreciating the culinary journey.

Incorporating Whole Foods into Your Diet

Now that we've highlighted the benefits of whole foods, let's explore how you can incorporate them into your daily diet:

1. Fruits and Vegetables: Aim to fill half your plate with a variety of colorful fruits and vegetables. These foods are rich in vitamins, minerals, and antioxidants. Experiment with different types and preparation methods to keep your meals exciting.

2. Whole Grains: Choose whole grains like brown rice, quinoa, oats, and whole wheat over refined grains. These grains provide sustained energy and dietary fiber, promoting digestive health.

3. Lean Proteins: Opt for lean sources of protein such as poultry, fish, legumes, and tofu. These options are lower in saturated fats and provide essential amino acids for muscle and tissue repair.

4. Healthy Fats: Incorporate sources of healthy fats like avocados, nuts, seeds, and olive oil. These fats support brain health, nutrient absorption, and overall well-being.

5. Dairy and Dairy Alternatives: If you consume dairy, choose low-fat or fat-free options. For those who prefer dairy alternatives, such as almond or soy milk, select unsweetened varieties.

6. Hydration: Don't forget about hydration. Water is an essential component of a mindful eating journey. Aim to drink plenty of water throughout the day to support digestion and overall health.

Mindful Meal Preparation

Incorporating whole foods into your meals can be an enjoyable and creative process. Mindful meal preparation involves selecting fresh ingredients, experimenting with flavors, and savoring the cooking process. When you're fully present in the kitchen, you'll find that mealtime becomes a celebration of nourishment and well-being.

As we continue our exploration of mindful eating and food choices, remember that whole foods are your allies in this journey. They not only provide nourishment for your body but also create an opportunity for mindfulness in every meal. So, let's embrace the power of nutritious, whole foods and make them a vibrant part of our mindful eating plate.

Understanding Food Labels Mindfully

Food labels serve as your compass in the world of packaged and processed foods. They provide essential information about the product's ingredients, nutritional content, and serving size. Here's how you can approach food labels mindfully:

1. Start with the Ingredient List:

- The ingredient list is your first stop when examining a food label. It lists the components of the product in descending order of quantity, with the most abundant ingredient listed first.
- Be on the lookout for whole and familiar ingredients. If you can't pronounce an ingredient or it sounds overly processed, it may be a sign to proceed with caution.

2. Check Serving Sizes:

- Serving sizes on food labels can be deceptive. Ensure you're comparing the serving size on the label to your actual portion size. This helps you avoid underestimating or overestimating the nutrients you're consuming.

3. Mindful of Macronutrients:

- Pay attention to the macronutrients—carbohydrates, proteins, and fats. Determine if the product aligns with your dietary preferences and needs.
- Remember that not all fats or carbohydrates are equal. Look for sources of healthy fats and complex carbohydrates in the ingredient list.

4. Beware of Added Sugars:

- Added sugars can be hiding under various names on food labels. Keep an eye out for terms like sucrose, high fructose corn syrup, and agave nectar. The closer added sugars are to the top of the ingredient list, the more sugar the product contains.

5. Mind the Sodium:

- Excessive sodium intake can contribute to health issues. Be mindful of the sodium content, especially in processed foods. Aim for products with lower sodium levels.

6. Fiber Matters:

- Dietary fiber is an essential component of a balanced diet. Look for products that provide a good source of dietary fiber, often found in whole grains, fruits, and vegetables.

7. Watch for Allergens:

- If you have allergies or sensitivities, be vigilant about allergen warnings on food labels. Manufacturers are required to clearly identify common allergens.

8. Seek Transparency:

- Choose products from companies that prioritize transparency and provide clear, honest information on their labels. Look for certifications like "Non-GMO" or "Organic" if they align with your values.

9. The Mindful Pause:

- Before placing an item in your cart, take a moment to pause and reflect. Ask yourself if the product supports your mindful eating goals and aligns with your values.

10. Less Is More:

- In the world of food labels, less is often more. Products with shorter ingredient lists tend to be less processed and closer to their whole food source.

Mindful Shopping and Label Reading

Incorporating mindfulness into your shopping routine can help you make intentional and health-conscious choices:

1. Create a List: Before heading to the store, make a list of the items you need. This reduces impulse purchases and keeps you focused on your mindful eating goals.

2. Shop the Perimeter: Whole foods like fruits, vegetables, lean proteins, and dairy products are typically found on the perimeter of the store. Spend more time in these sections.

3. Minimize Packaged Foods: Aim to fill your cart with a majority of whole, unprocessed foods. Limit your purchases of highly processed items.

4. Avoid Shopping Hungry: Shopping on an empty stomach can lead to impulsive and less mindful choices. Eat a small meal or snack before shopping.

By understanding food labels mindfully and adopting conscious shopping habits, you empower yourself to make food choices that align with your values and support your mindful eating journey. Remember that each choice you make is an opportunity to nourish your body and enhance your overall well-being.

Mindful Dining Out: Tips for a Positive Experience

1. **Plan Ahead:**
   - Before heading to the restaurant, take a look at the menu online if available. This allows you to preselect options that align with your dietary preferences and mindful eating goals.
2. **Listen to Your Body:**

- When you arrive at the restaurant, take a moment to check in with your body. Are you genuinely hungry, or are you eating out of habit or social pressure? Make choices based on your true hunger cues.

3. **Mindful Ordering:**
   - Choose dishes that include a balance of protein, vegetables, and whole grains if possible. Look for keywords like "grilled," "baked," or "steamed" rather than "fried" or "crispy."

4. **Portion Control:**
   - Restaurant portions are often larger than what you need. Consider sharing an entrée with a friend or requesting a to-go container at the beginning of the meal to save half for later.

5. **Savor the Experience:**
   - Take your time to eat and savor each bite. Engage all your senses and appreciate the flavors, textures, and aromas of the food.

6. **Mindful Eating Techniques:**
   - Use mindful eating techniques like eating with utensils instead of your hands, taking small bites, and putting your fork down between bites. These practices help you eat more slowly and mindfully.

7. **Hydration:**
   - Opt for water or herbal tea as your beverage of choice. Avoid sugary sodas and excessive alcohol, which can add empty calories to your meal.

8. **Special Requests:**
   - Don't hesitate to make special requests, such as asking for sauces or dressings on the side or substituting ingredients to meet your dietary needs.

9. **Dessert Deliberation:**
   - If you're considering dessert, share it with others at the table. Sharing allows you to enjoy a sweet treat without overindulging.

10. **Practice Gratitude:**

- Take a moment of gratitude before and after your meal. Reflect on the experience and appreciate the nourishment you've received.

Mindful Social Dining

Eating out often involves social interactions, which can sometimes lead to less mindful choices. Here's how to maintain mindfulness in social dining situations:

1. **Communicate Your Intentions:**
   - Let your dining companions know that you value mindful eating and your health. They may be more understanding and supportive of your choices.
2. **Lead by Example:**
   - Showcase mindful eating habits to your friends and family. Your mindful choices may inspire them to be more conscious about their own eating habits.
3. **Respect Others' Choices:**
   - While it's important to communicate your intentions, also respect the choices of others. Everyone has their own relationship with food, and judgment-free support goes a long way.

Mindful Reflection After the Meal

After your dining experience, take a moment to reflect mindfully:

1. **How Do You Feel?:**
   - Tune in to how your body feels after the meal. Are you comfortably satisfied, or do you feel overly full or uncomfortable? Reflecting on these sensations can guide future choices.
2. **Emotional Well-Being:**
   - Pay attention to your emotional state. Did you enjoy the social aspect of dining out? Did you feel guilty or anxious

about your food choices? Mindful reflection can help you understand your emotional relationship with food.

Remember that dining out is meant to be an enjoyable experience. By approaching it mindfully and making conscious choices, you can savor the flavors, appreciate the company, and nourish your body and soul simultaneously. Enjoy your restaurant meals as a part of your mindful eating journey, making each dining experience a positive and satisfying one.

Mindful Recipes: Nourishing Body and Soul

1. **Mango and Avocado Salad with Lime Dressing:**
   - This refreshing salad combines the sweetness of ripe mangoes with the creaminess of avocados. Drizzle it with a zesty lime dressing for a burst of flavor. Each bite is a celebration of vibrant colors and contrasting textures.

2. **Quinoa and Vegetable Stir-Fry:**
   - Stir-fries are a quick and versatile way to enjoy a variety of vegetables and proteins. Prepare a colorful quinoa and vegetable stir-fry with your choice of tofu, shrimp, or chicken. Customize the sauce to your taste, and savor the medley of flavors in every bite.

3. **Mediterranean Chickpea Bowl:**
   - This Mediterranean-inspired bowl features chickpeas as the star ingredient. Combine them with fresh cucumbers, cherry tomatoes, olives, and feta cheese. Top it off with a drizzle of olive oil and a sprinkle of fresh herbs for a taste of the Mediterranean.

4. **Baked Sweet Potato Fries:**
   - Craving something crispy? Try baking sweet potato fries for a healthy and satisfying snack or side dish. Season them with your favorite herbs and spices for an extra kick of flavor.

5. **Coconut Chia Pudding with Berries:**
   - For a delightful dessert or breakfast option, prepare coconut chia pudding topped with a colorful array of fresh berries.

The creamy, coconut-infused pudding pairs perfectly with the natural sweetness of the berries.

Mindful Meal Planning Ideas

1. **Theme Nights:**
   - Incorporate theme nights into your meal planning. For example, have a "Meatless Monday" where you explore vegetarian or vegan recipes. "Taco Tuesday" can feature a variety of taco fillings and toppings.

2. **Batch Cooking:**
   - Save time and reduce food waste by batch cooking staples like grains, beans, and roasted vegetables. These can serve as the base for multiple meals throughout the week.

3. **Mindful Snacking:**
   - Plan for mindful snacks by having a variety of healthy options readily available. Cut up fresh vegetables, prepare yogurt parfaits with fruit and granola, or have a small handful of nuts on hand.

4. **Balanced Plates:**
   - Aim for balanced meals that include a protein source, a generous serving of vegetables, and a portion of whole grains or starchy vegetables. This ensures you're nourishing your body with a variety of nutrients.

5. **Mindful Leftovers:**
   - Transform leftovers into new and exciting dishes. For example, last night's roasted chicken can become today's chicken salad or chicken quesadillas.

Cultivating Mindfulness in the Kitchen

While preparing these meals, practice mindfulness in the kitchen:

1. **Sensory Engagement:**
   - Engage your senses while cooking. Feel the texture of

ingredients, inhale the aromas, and taste as you go. Cooking becomes a sensory experience that enhances your connection with food.

2. **Mindful Chopping:**
   - When chopping vegetables or ingredients, focus on the rhythm of your knife and the sounds it makes. Be fully present in the act of chopping, free from distractions.

3. **Gratitude and Appreciation:**
   - As you cook and enjoy your meals, express gratitude for the nourishment and pleasure that food provides. Appreciate the effort and love you put into preparing your dishes.

Inspiring Your Mindful Eating Journey

These recipes and meal planning ideas are not just about satisfying hunger—they're about cultivating a deeper connection with the food you eat. They encourage you to savor the present moment, appreciate the ingredients, and celebrate the nourishment of your body and soul.

So, roll up your sleeves, put on your apron, and embark on this mindful cooking adventure. Let your kitchen become a place of mindfulness, creativity, and joy as you explore the wonderful world of mindful recipes and meal planning. Enjoy every bite and relish the journey!

Chapter 8: Mindful Eating for Mental Health

Welcome to Chapter 8, where we explore the profound connection between mindful eating and mental health. Your emotional well-being is just as important as your physical health, and what you eat plays a crucial role in shaping your mood, thoughts, and overall mental state. In this chapter, we will uncover the fascinating interplay between your diet and your mental health, and how embracing mindful eating can be a game-changer.

How's your mood today? Your diet might have something to do with it.

Ever noticed how certain foods can affect your mood? It's not just a coincidence; there's a profound connection between what you eat and how you feel. Let's take a closer look:

1. Nutrient-Rich Foods for Mood Enhancement:

- Nutrient-dense foods, particularly those rich in vitamins, minerals, and antioxidants, play a crucial role in supporting mental health. For example, foods high in omega-3 fatty acids, such as fatty fish like salmon and walnuts, are known to promote brain health and reduce symptoms of depression.

2. The Impact of Sugar and Processed Foods:

- On the flip side, excessive sugar and highly processed foods can lead to mood swings, energy crashes, and feelings of irritability. These foods may provide a temporary spike in mood, but they are often followed by a crash, leaving you feeling worse than before.

3. The Gut-Brain Connection:

- Emerging research has revealed the importance of gut health in influencing mood. A balanced and diverse diet that includes fiber-rich foods, probiotics, and prebiotics can foster a healthy gut microbiome, positively impacting mental health.

4. Mindful Eating Practices and Emotional Well-Being:

- Mindful eating goes beyond the types of foods you consume; it also encompasses how you eat. When you practice mindful eating, you're more attuned to your body's hunger and fullness cues. This awareness can help you avoid overeating or seeking comfort in food when you're not truly hungry.

5. The Role of Hydration:

- Dehydration can lead to mood swings and decreased cognitive function. Ensuring you're well-hydrated throughout the day is a simple yet effective way to support your mental well-being.

Mindful Eating for Emotional Well-Being

Now, let's explore how you can incorporate mindful eating practices to enhance your emotional well-being:

1. Recognize Emotional Eating:

- Chapter 8 delves into the significance of recognizing emotional eating. Are you eating because you're genuinely hungry, or are you using food to cope with stress, sadness, or boredom? Mindful eating encourages you to identify emotional triggers for eating and develop healthier coping mechanisms.

2. Slow Down and Savor:

- Mindful eating practices promote slowing down the pace of your meal, allowing you to savor each bite fully. This practice can create a sense of satisfaction and pleasure, which can positively impact your mood.

3. Choose Mood-Supportive Foods:

- Chapter 8 discusses how you can make mindful choices about the foods you consume to support your mental health. Nutrient-rich foods like fruits, vegetables, whole grains, and lean proteins provide the essential vitamins and minerals your brain needs to function optimally.

4. Mindful Snacking:

- Delving into mindful snacking, we'll explore how to choose snacks that boost your mood and energy levels without compromising your overall well-being.

As we journey through Chapter 8, you'll discover the profound influence that mindful eating can have on your mental health. Your diet is not just about fueling your body; it's also about nourishing your mind and emotions. So, let's delve deeper into the ways you can harness the power of mindful eating to support your mental well-being and foster a happier, healthier you.

Understanding the Stress-Food Connection

Stress and food are intertwined in complex ways. For some, stress can lead to overeating or making unhealthy food choices as a way to cope. Others might experience a loss of appetite or neglect nourishing themselves when stress takes over. Mindful eating offers a path to break free from these patterns and find balance.

1. Awareness of Stress Triggers:

- Mindful eating begins with self-awareness. Take time to recognize your stress triggers. Is it work-related pressure, relationship challenges, or external circumstances? Understanding what's causing your stress is the first step in addressing it mindfully.

2. Mindful Stress Response:

- Instead of turning to food automatically when stressed, practice pausing. When you feel the urge to eat in response to stress, pause and check in with yourself. Are you physically hungry, or is this emotional hunger? This simple act of mindfulness can help you choose a more constructive response.

3. Mindful Breathing:

- Deep, mindful breathing is a potent stress-reduction tool. When you're stressed, your breath tends to become shallow and rapid. By consciously slowing down your breath and taking deep, intentional breaths, you activate the body's relaxation response, reducing stress and anxiety.

4. Eating with Presence:

- When you do eat, do it with full presence. Avoid eating in front of screens or while multitasking. Instead, sit down at a table, savor each bite, and engage your senses fully. Notice the textures, flavors, and aromas of your food.

5. Use Food as Nourishment:

- Embrace food as a source of nourishment for your body and mind. Choose foods that provide sustained energy and support overall well-being. Incorporate a balance of vegetables, whole grains, lean proteins, and healthy fats into your meals.

6. Mindful Portion Control:

- Practice portion control mindfully. Overeating can lead to physical discomfort, which can exacerbate stress. By paying attention to your body's cues for hunger and fullness, you can avoid overindulging.

7. Mindful Eating Rituals:

- Create mindful eating rituals to help you manage stress. Consider starting or ending your meal with a moment of gratitude, expressing appreciation for the nourishment your meal provides.

8. Seek Support:

- If you find that stress and anxiety significantly impact your eating habits, consider seeking support from a mental health professional or counselor. They can provide guidance and strategies to manage stress in a healthy way.

Mindful Eating as a Lifelong Skill

Remember that mindful eating is not a quick fix but a lifelong skill that can positively impact your relationship with food and your overall well-being. By approaching food and eating with mindfulness, you can reduce anxiety and stress, and cultivate a deeper sense of peace and balance in your life. So, as you continue your mindful eating journey, use these practices to help you navigate the challenges of stress with grace and resilience.

1. The Mindful Pause:

- The mindful pause is a simple yet potent practice. Throughout your day, set aside a few moments to pause and be fully present. Whether you're sipping your morning coffee, taking a break at work, or waiting in line, use this time to bring your attention to your breath. Inhale deeply, exhale slowly, and notice the sensations in your body and your surroundings. This practice can help you recenter and reduce stress.

2. Body Scan Meditation:

- Find a comfortable, quiet space to sit or lie down. Close your eyes and bring your attention to your body. Starting from your toes, slowly scan your body's sensations, inch by inch, all the way up to the top of your head. Notice any areas of tension or discomfort, and simply observe them without judgment. The body scan can help you release physical tension and cultivate body awareness.

3. Gratitude Journaling:

- Keep a gratitude journal by your bedside. Each night, jot down three things you're grateful for. These can be simple pleasures, moments of kindness, or anything that brings you joy. Cultivating gratitude can shift your focus toward positivity and improve your overall mental well-being.

4. Mindful Breathing for Stress Reduction:

- During moments of stress, practice mindful breathing. Find a quiet space, sit comfortably, and close your eyes. Take a deep breath in through your nose for a count of four, hold for a count of four, and exhale through your mouth for a count of four. Repeat this cycle for several breaths. This exercise calms the nervous system and reduces stress hormones.

5. Mindful Walking:

- Incorporate mindfulness into your daily walks. As you walk, pay attention to the sensation of each step, the feeling of the ground beneath your feet, and the movement of your body. Notice the sights, sounds, and smells around you. This practice can turn a simple walk into a meditative experience.

6. Loving-Kindness Meditation:

- Dedicate time to loving-kindness meditation. Sit in a quiet space, close your eyes, and silently repeat phrases like, "May I be happy. May I be healthy. May I be safe. May I live with ease." Extend these wishes to yourself, loved ones, acquaintances, and even those you may have conflicts with. This practice fosters compassion and empathy, promoting positive mental well-being.

7. Mindful Eating Meditation:

- While enjoying a meal, practice a mindful eating meditation. As you take each bite, savor the flavors, textures, and aromas of your food.

Notice the physical sensations of chewing and swallowing. Put down your utensils between bites, and focus solely on the act of eating. This practice not only enhances your appreciation of food but also promotes mindful awareness.

8. Breathing Space:

- When you're feeling overwhelmed, take a "breathing space" break. Find a quiet spot, sit comfortably, and follow these three steps:

- **Gather Your Attention:** Close your eyes, take a few deep breaths, and notice what's happening within and around you.
- **The Present Moment:** Shift your attention to the sensations of your breath. Follow the breath as it enters and leaves your body.
- **Expanding Awareness:** Gradually expand your awareness to your body, thoughts, and emotions. Notice without judgment. This exercise helps you regain a sense of calm and perspective.

These practical mindfulness exercises are like mental tools you can keep in your toolbox, ready to use whenever you need them. Regular practice can help you build resilience, reduce stress, and boost your mental well-being. So, as you embark on your mindful eating journey, remember that mindfulness extends beyond the plate and into every aspect of your life, enriching your experience and nurturing your mental health.

Transformative Stories of Mindful Eating

"In the realm of mindful eating, personal stories often shine the brightest. These are tales of transformation, of individuals who, like you, embarked on a journey to explore the profound connection between food and emotions."

1. Sarah's Journey to Overcoming Emotional Eating:

- Sarah, a 34-year-old professional, had struggled with emotional eating for years. Stress at work and personal challenges often led her to find comfort in unhealthy foods. Through mindfulness practices, Sarah learned to identify her emotional triggers and respond to them mindfully. She discovered that savoring a piece of dark chocolate mindfully provided the same comfort without the guilt. Her journey showcases the power of mindful eating in breaking free from emotional food cravings.

2. Mark's Battle with Depression and Nutritional Healing:

- Mark had battled depression for much of his life. He often turned to fast food and sugary snacks as a form of self-medication. A chance encounter with mindful eating practices opened his eyes to the impact of his diet on his mood. Mark began incorporating more whole foods, such as fruits, vegetables, and lean proteins, into his meals. Over time, he noticed a significant improvement in his mood and a reduction in depressive symptoms. His story illustrates how dietary changes can complement mental health treatments.

3. Maria's Journey to Rediscovering Joy in Eating:

- Maria, a 45-year-old mother of two, had lost the joy of eating due to years of dieting and restrictive eating patterns. Mindful eating helped her reconnect with the pleasures of food. She learned to appreciate the colors, textures, and flavors of each meal. Rediscovering the joy of eating without guilt or judgment brought a sense of fulfillment back into her life. Maria's story emphasizes the importance of savoring food as a source of happiness.

4. James' Path to Reducing Anxiety with Food Choices:

- James, a young adult, had battled anxiety for years. He noticed that his anxiety often worsened after consuming caffeine and processed foods. Through mindful eating practices, he began to make more informed food choices. By reducing his intake of caffeine and processed snacks and incorporating more calming foods like herbal teas and leafy greens, James experienced a significant reduction in anxiety symptoms. His story highlights the role of diet in managing anxiety.

The Science Behind Diet and Mental Health

"Beyond personal narratives, the science behind the diet-mental health connection offers valuable insights into how the foods we consume impact our emotional well-being."

1. Nutrients that Nourish the Brain:

- The brain requires a variety of nutrients, including omega-3 fatty acids, antioxidants, vitamins, and minerals, to function optimally. These nutrients are found in abundance in whole foods like fish, nuts, berries, leafy greens, and whole grains. Research suggests that a diet rich in these brain-boosting nutrients can enhance mood, reduce symptoms of depression, and support overall mental health.

2. Gut Health and Mood:

- The gut-brain connection is a burgeoning field of research. Emerging studies have shown that the health of your gut microbiome, the trillions of microorganisms living in your digestive system, can influence your mood and mental health. Consuming a diet rich in fiber, prebiotics, and probiotics can promote a healthy gut microbiome, potentially reducing the risk of mood disorders.

3. The Impact of Sugar and Processed Foods:

- High sugar and highly processed diets have been linked to mood swings, increased risk of depression, and heightened anxiety. The rapid spikes and crashes in blood sugar levels that follow the consumption of these foods can negatively affect mood and overall mental well-being.

4. Mindful Eating as a Stress Reduction Tool:

- Mindful eating practices, as we've explored throughout this book, can reduce stress by promoting relaxation responses in the body. The act of mindful eating encourages you to savor each bite, creating a sense of satisfaction and tranquility.

5. Diet as Complementary to Mental Health Treatments:

- While diet alone may not be a substitute for professional mental health treatment, it can be a valuable complement. Many individuals, as showcased in the stories above, have found relief from symptoms of anxiety, depression, and emotional eating by making mindful dietary choices alongside therapy or medication.

As you continue your journey into the world of mindful eating, remember that your relationship with food is deeply intertwined with your emotional well-being. By exploring these personal stories and the scientific underpinnings, you gain a deeper understanding of the profound impact that food choices can have on your mental health. Embrace the knowledge that you have the power to transform your relationship with food and, in turn, your emotional well-being.

Chapter 9: Mindful Eating in Social Situations

Welcome to Chapter 9, where we'll explore the art of mindful eating in social situations. We understand that social gatherings, parties, and events can present unique challenges when it comes to maintaining your mindful eating practice. However, fear not, for we're here to provide you with effective strategies to navigate these tricky waters and stay true to your mindful eating journey.

The Challenges of Being the Mindful Eater at Social Events

"Picture this: You're at a bustling social event, surrounded by friends, family, or colleagues, and the tables are laden with an array of tempting dishes and appetizers. The atmosphere is lively, and it's easy to get caught up in the excitement. But as a mindful eater, you face specific challenges that require a delicate balance between enjoying the social experience and honoring your commitment to mindful eating."

1. The Temptation of Mindless Eating:

- In social situations, it's all too common to mindlessly munch on appetizers or snacks as you engage in conversations or wait for the main meal. These unconscious eating habits can lead to overindulgence and disrupt your mindful eating practice.

2. Peer Pressure and Food Choices:

- Social gatherings often involve peer pressure when it comes to food choices. Friends or family may encourage you to try certain dishes or indulge in desserts. Balancing social expectations with your mindful eating principles can be challenging.

3. Fast-Paced Eating:

- The fast-paced nature of social events can lead to hurried eating. You might find yourself rushing through your meal or not fully savoring the flavors and textures of the dishes.

4. Emotional Eating Triggers:

- Social events can evoke various emotions, from excitement and happiness to stress or anxiety. Emotional triggers can lead to impulsive eating or seeking comfort in food.

5. Staying Present in Social Interactions:

- Maintaining meaningful connections with others at social gatherings while also staying present in your eating experience requires a delicate balance.

Strategies for Mindful Eating in Social Situations

Now, let's explore effective strategies to help you overcome these challenges and practice mindful eating during social events:

1. Set Clear Intentions:

- Before attending a social gathering, set clear intentions for your mindful eating practice. Remind yourself of your commitment to nourishing your body and savoring the flavors of food mindfully.

2. Mindful Pre-Eating Ritual:

- Take a few moments to practice mindfulness before you start eating. Focus on your breath, center yourself, and cultivate awareness of your surroundings and the people you're with.

3. Choose Mindfully:

- When faced with an array of food choices, take a mindful moment to decide what truly appeals to you. Select dishes that align with your mindful eating values and preferences.

4. Practice Portion Control:

- Be conscious of portion sizes. Serve yourself moderate portions and, if possible, use smaller plates to help control the amount you eat.

5. Savor Each Bite:

- Slow down and savor each bite. Pay attention to the colors, textures, and flavors of the food. Engage your senses fully in the eating experience.

6. Stay Hydrated:

- Drink water throughout the event to stay hydrated. Sometimes, thirst can be mistaken for hunger, leading to unnecessary snacking.

7. Manage Peer Pressure Gracefully:

- Politely and confidently decline food offerings if they don't align with your mindful eating goals. Communicate your commitment to your well-being without judgment or criticism.

8. Be Mindful of Emotional Eating:

- Be aware of your emotional state during social events. If you find yourself reaching for food in response to stress or other emotions, pause and consider alternative coping strategies, such as deep breathing or engaging in a conversation.

9. Balance Social Interaction and Eating:

- Strike a balance between social interactions and mindful eating. Engage in conversations, laughter, and connection with others while also savoring your food.

10. Express Gratitude:

- At the end of the meal, express gratitude for the nourishment and the company. Gratitude can deepen your mindful eating practice and enhance your overall well-being.

By implementing these strategies, you can navigate social situations with confidence and grace, all while staying true to your commitment to mindful eating. Remember that mindful eating is not about deprivation but about fostering a harmonious relationship with food and enjoying the pleasures of eating in a mindful and balanced way.

Learning to Say No Gracefully to Tempting, Unhealthy Offers

"In the realm of mindful eating, saying no gracefully can be a valuable skill. It allows you to make choices that align with your well-being while maintaining respect for yourself and others. Let's explore how to navigate tempting, unhealthy offers with confidence and mindfulness."

1. The Power of Polite Declines:

- One of the most effective ways to say no gracefully is through polite and respectful declines. When offered tempting, unhealthy foods, you can respond with a simple, "No, thank you," or "I appreciate the offer, but I'm going to pass."

2. Express Your Priorities:

- If someone insists or questions your decision, you can gently express your priorities. For example, "I'm focusing on nourishing my body in a way that makes me feel my best," or "I've already enjoyed some delicious food, and I'm satisfied for now."

3. Redirect the Focus:

- Shift the conversation away from food by redirecting the focus. Engage in a different topic or compliment the host on their hospitality. Redirecting the conversation can create a positive atmosphere and minimize pressure.

4. Offer a Future Date:

- If the temptation is related to a special treat or dessert, you can gracefully decline by suggesting a future date. Say something like, "That looks amazing! I'll have to try it next time," or "I'm saving room for now, but I'd love to taste it another time."

5. Mindful Self-Compassion:

- Practice mindful self-compassion when saying no. Remember that your well-being is a priority, and making choices that honor your health is an act of self-love. Avoid self-judgment or guilt for declining tempting offers.

6. Non-Verbal Communication:

- Sometimes, a simple non-verbal response can convey your choice gracefully. A warm smile, a gentle shake of the head, or placing your hand over your heart can communicate your decision without words.

7. Be Firm but Kind:

- If the offers persist, it's okay to be firm in your decision while remaining kind and respectful. Say, "I appreciate your kindness, but I've made a conscious choice to stick to my mindful eating plan."

8. Have a Support Buddy:

- If you're at a social event with a supportive friend or family member who understands your mindful eating goals, enlist their help. They can provide support by backing up your choices and helping you navigate challenging situations.

9. Practice Mindful Awareness:

- Stay mindful of your body's cues and your personal goals. When faced with tempting offers, take a moment to check in with yourself. Ask, "Am I physically hungry, or is this a craving influenced by external factors?"

10. Be Grateful and Appreciative:

- Always express gratitude and appreciation for the offer and the thoughtfulness behind it. Saying no gracefully doesn't mean rejecting kindness. Instead, it's about making choices that align with your values and well-being.

Remember, saying no gracefully is not about rejecting others or their offerings but about making choices that support your health and mindfulness journey. By practicing these strategies, you can navigate tempting, unhealthy offers with confidence and respect for yourself and those around you.

Your Survival Guide for Parties and Family Gatherings

"Social gatherings with friends and family can be delightful, but they can also pose challenges for mindful eaters. That's why we've prepared a survival guide to help you navigate these occasions while staying true to your mindful eating journey."

1. Plan Ahead:

- Before attending a party or family gathering, take a moment to plan your approach. Consider what foods will likely be served and how you can align your choices with your mindful eating goals.

2. Eat Mindfully Beforehand:

- Have a balanced and satisfying meal before the event to curb excessive hunger. When you arrive, you'll be less likely to indulge in unhealthy options out of sheer hunger.

3. Communicate Your Preferences:

- If you're comfortable doing so, communicate your mindful eating preferences with the host or organizer. They may appreciate knowing your dietary preferences or restrictions in advance.

4. Survey the Spread:

- When you arrive, take a moment to survey the food options available. Identify dishes that align with your mindful eating principles and focus on those.

5. Portion Control:

- Use smaller plates and practice portion control. Start with smaller servings, and if you'd like more, you can always return for seconds.

6. Savor Each Bite:

- Eat slowly and savor each bite. Engage your senses by paying attention to the colors, textures, and flavors of the food.

7. Stay Hydrated:

- Drink water throughout the event to stay hydrated. Sometimes, thirst can be mistaken for hunger, leading to unnecessary snacking.

8. Practice Mindful Conversations:

- Engage in meaningful conversations with friends and family. Being present in these interactions can help reduce mindless snacking.

9. Bring a Mindful Dish:

- Consider bringing a dish that aligns with your mindful eating values. This way, you'll have a guaranteed healthy option available.

10. Mindful Indulgence: - If there's a special treat you'd like to enjoy, do so mindfully. Take a small portion, savor it fully, and appreciate the experience.

11. Manage Social Pressure: - If others encourage you to eat more or indulge, politely and confidently express your preferences. Remember, you're making choices that align with your well-being.

12. Be Compassionate: - Practice self-compassion and avoid self-judgment. If you deviate from your mindful eating plan, acknowledge it without guilt and refocus on your goals.

13. Support System: - If possible, have a supportive friend or family member accompany you who understands your mindful eating journey. They can provide encouragement and support.

14. Mindful Departure: - When it's time to leave the gathering, reflect on your experience. Celebrate your mindful choices and consider what you learned from the event.

15. Gratitude and Connection: - Focus on the joy of connecting with loved ones rather than solely on the food. Express gratitude for the experience and the people you shared it with.

By following these guidelines, you can navigate parties and family gatherings with confidence, enjoying both the company of loved ones and the mindful choices that support your well-being. Remember that mindful eating is a journey, and every choice you make is an opportunity to nurture a healthier relationship with food.

Real-Life Stories of Mindful Socializing

"In the world of mindful eating, real-life stories often serve as beacons of inspiration. These stories are a testament to the power of mindfulness even in the midst of socializing and gatherings. Let's dive into the experiences of individuals who have managed to keep their mindfulness intact while enjoying social occasions."

1. Sarah's Mindful Cocktail Hour:

- Sarah, a social butterfly known for hosting vibrant gatherings, discovered the art of mindful cocktail hours. Instead of indulging in numerous drinks, she began to savor a single, well-crafted cocktail. By paying attention to each sip and engaging in meaningful conversations, Sarah found that she could enjoy the social aspect of gatherings without overindulging. Her friends soon followed suit, and mindful cocktail hours became a cherished tradition among her circle.

2. Mark's Family Reunion Feast:

- Mark, who values mindful eating for its health benefits, faced a significant challenge at his family's annual reunion feast, where rich, indulgent dishes were the norm. Instead of resisting the delicious temptations, Mark decided to approach the event with an open heart and mind. He filled his plate with a variety of foods, each chosen mindfully, and savored every bite. Mark's family was inspired by his approach and began to focus more on the experience of sharing meals together rather than the quantity of food consumed.

3. Maria's Thanksgiving Transformation:

- Maria had always associated Thanksgiving with overeating and discomfort. Determined to break this pattern, she introduced mindfulness to her family's Thanksgiving celebration. She encouraged everyone to express gratitude for the meal and share their reflections on the year. As a result, the meal became more about connection and thankfulness than excess. The family even started a tradition of taking a mindful walk after dinner, appreciating the beauty of nature and each other's company.

4. James' Mindful Picnic Adventure:

- James, an avid nature enthusiast, discovered that mindfulness could extend to outdoor gatherings as well. He organized mindful picnics with friends, where they would bring healthy, locally sourced foods and eat while immersed in the beauty of the natural surroundings. These picnics became an opportunity to connect with nature, nourish their bodies, and strengthen their friendships. James and his friends found that mindful picnics allowed them to enjoy socializing without the typical indulgence of unhealthy snacks.

Creating Supportive Social Environments for Mindful Eating

"In addition to real-life stories of mindful socializing, it's important to explore ways to create supportive social environments that encourage mindful eating. Here are some tips to foster a mindful atmosphere during gatherings with friends and family:"

1. Lead by Example:

- Be a mindful eater and lead by example. Your mindful choices can inspire others to approach meals with greater awareness.

2. Share Your Journey:

- Communicate your mindful eating journey with friends and family. Explain the benefits it has brought to your life and why it's important to you.

3. Collaborative Cooking:

- Encourage collaborative cooking during gatherings. Cooking together can create a sense of connection and mindfulness as you prepare and savor the meal.

4. Mindful Rituals:

- Introduce mindful rituals into social events, such as a moment of gratitude before eating or a mindful breathing exercise to center everyone.

5. Limit Distractions:

- Minimize distractions like television or smartphones during meals. Create an environment that encourages conversation and connection.

6. Provide Healthy Options:

- When hosting, offer a variety of healthy and delicious options. This ensures that mindful eating is accessible to all, regardless of dietary preferences.

7. Respect Individual Choices:

- Respect the choices of others, even if they differ from your own mindful eating practices. Encourage an atmosphere of acceptance and non-judgment.

8. Engage in Mindful Activities:

- Incorporate mindful activities into gatherings, such as mindful walks, meditation sessions, or even group yoga.

9. Encourage Conversation:

- Foster meaningful conversations that go beyond small talk. Encourage discussions about well-being, personal growth, and gratitude.

10. Reflect and Share: - After the gathering, take a moment to reflect on the experience with your friends and family. Share what you enjoyed most and how the mindful aspects enriched the event.

Creating a supportive social environment that encourages mindful eating can have a positive impact not only on your own well-being but also on the well-being of those you care about. By incorporating mindfulness into social occasions, you can strengthen connections, deepen your appreciation for food, and collectively embark on a journey of holistic well-being.

Chapter 10: Sustaining a Mindful Eating Lifestyle

Welcome to Chapter 10, where we'll explore the art of sustaining a mindful eating lifestyle. As you've journeyed through this book, you've gained valuable insights into the practice of mindful eating and its transformative potential. Now, let's recap the key takeaways from our journey so far.

Recap of Our Mindful Eating Journey:

Throughout this book, we've embarked on a transformative journey into the world of mindful eating. Here's a brief recap of the key concepts and practices you've encountered:

1. Understanding Mindful Eating:

- Mindful eating is a holistic approach to food and nourishment rooted in mindfulness meditation. It involves cultivating a deep awareness of your relationship with food, your body, and the act of eating itself.

2. The Importance of Being Mindful:

- Mindful eating is not a luxury but a necessity for overall well-being. It offers a path to break free from unhealthy eating habits, reduce mealtime stress, and savor the joys of nourishing your body and soul.

3. The Mind-Body Connection:

- Your mind and body are interconnected, and this connection profoundly influences your eating habits. Mindful eating helps you become aware of emotional triggers and the importance of responding to your body's hunger and fullness cues.

4. Breaking Unhealthy Patterns:

- Mindful eating empowers you to untangle complex emotional relationships with food and differentiate between physical hunger and emotional cravings. It's about savoring foods you love in moderation without guilt or judgment.

5. Recognizing Hunger and Fullness:

- Learning to recognize physical hunger cues is essential for mindful eating. It enables you to eat when you're hungry and stop when you're satisfied, promoting a balanced relationship with food.

6. Mindful Eating for Weight Management:

- Research shows that mindful eating can support weight loss and help break free from dieting cycles. It emphasizes the importance of making conscious choices and listening to your body's signals.

7. The Emotional Connection to Food:

- Emotional eating is a common challenge, but mindfulness can help you conquer it. By recognizing emotional triggers and responding with mindfulness, you can develop healthier coping strategies.

8. Mindful Eating in a Fast-Paced World:

- Mindful eating is achievable even in today's hectic lifestyles. Practical tips, stress reduction techniques, and on-the-go strategies empower you to incorporate mindfulness into your daily routines.

9. Mindful Eating for Improved Digestion:

- Mindful eating can enhance digestion by promoting slower, more relaxed meals and better food choices. It's about nourishing your body with intention and care.

10. Mindful Eating and Food Choices: - Mindfulness guides your food choices toward nutritious, whole foods. It helps you navigate food labels, make mindful decisions when dining out, and even inspires you with delicious recipes.

11. Mindful Eating for Mental Health: - Your diet plays a significant role in your mood and mental well-being. Mindful eating can reduce anxiety and stress, and practical exercises can boost your mental health.

12. Mindful Eating in Social Situations: - Social gatherings and family events can present challenges, but with strategies like setting intentions, practicing mindful conversations, and expressing gratitude, you can navigate them gracefully.

13. Real-Life Stories and Supportive Environments: - Real-life stories of individuals who've maintained mindfulness while socializing serve as inspiration. Creating supportive social environments encourages mindful eating among friends and family.

Sustaining Your Mindful Eating Journey:

Now that you've absorbed the wisdom of mindful eating, it's time to focus on sustaining this valuable practice in your life. Here are some key principles to help you maintain a mindful eating lifestyle:

1. Consistency is Key:

- Mindful eating is a skill that deepens with practice. Consistency in your mindful eating habits is essential for long-term success.

2. Mindful Moments:

- Incorporate mindful moments throughout your day. Pause and take a few deep breaths before eating or making food choices.

3. Mindful Eating Communities:

- Join or create mindful eating communities. Sharing your journey with like-minded individuals can provide support and motivation.

4. Mindful Shopping:

- Extend mindfulness to your grocery shopping. Choose fresh, whole foods mindfully and read labels with awareness.

5. Continued Learning:

- Stay curious and open to continued learning about mindful eating. There's always more to discover and explore on this transformative journey.

6. Self-Compassion:

- Practice self-compassion on your mindful eating journey. Be gentle with yourself, and remember that it's okay to have moments of mindlessness.

7. Flexibility and Adaptability:

- Be flexible and adaptable in different situations. Mindful eating doesn't require perfection; it's about progress and growth.

8. Reflection and Gratitude:

- Reflect on your mindful eating experiences and express gratitude for the positive changes it has brought to your life.

As you continue your mindful eating journey, remember that it's a lifelong practice that can bring joy, health, and fulfillment. By consistently applying mindfulness to your relationship with food, you'll nurture a deep connection to nourishment, well-being, and the profound wisdom of your own body.

Step-by-Step Guidance for Daily Mindful Eating

"Congratulations on reaching this point in your mindful eating journey! You're now equipped with a profound understanding of the principles and practices that can transform your relationship with food. In this section, we provide you with step-by-step guidance on how to seamlessly weave mindful eating into your daily life."

Step 1: Morning Mindfulness

- Start your day with a moment of mindfulness. As you prepare breakfast or your morning beverage, take a few deep breaths. Engage your senses by appreciating the aromas and colors of your food or drink.

Step 2: Mindful Meal Preparation

- Extend mindfulness to meal preparation. As you gather ingredients and cook, focus on the textures, smells, and sounds of cooking. Consider the nourishment these foods will provide your body.

Step 3: Setting Intentions

- Before each meal or snack, set a mindful intention. Ask yourself how you want to feel after eating. This simple act can guide your choices and bring awareness to your eating experience.

Step 4: Mindful Eating Space

- Create a mindful eating space free from distractions. Turn off screens, put away electronic devices, and set the table with care. This environment encourages focused eating.

Step 5: Engage Your Senses

- As you begin to eat, engage your senses fully. Notice the colors, textures, and aromas of your food. Take small, deliberate bites, and chew slowly, savoring each mouthful.

Step 6: Be Present

- Be fully present during the meal. If your mind starts to wander, gently bring it back to the act of eating. Avoid multitasking or rushing through your meal.

Step 7: Check-In with Hunger

- Pause during the meal to check in with your hunger. Are you still hungry, or are you satisfied? This practice helps you eat in alignment with your body's needs.

Step 8: Mindful Conversations

- If you're dining with others, engage in mindful conversations. Share thoughts and stories related to the meal. Being present with loved ones enhances the mealtime experience.

Step 9: Mindful Post-Meal Ritual

- After finishing your meal, take a few moments to reflect on the experience. Consider how the food nourished you and express gratitude for the nourishment.

Step 10: Daily Mindful Moments - Throughout the day, practice mindful moments related to food. When snacking, pause to appreciate the flavors. When making food choices, consider the impact on your well-being.

Step 11: Self-Compassion - Embrace self-compassion on your mindful eating journey. If you have moments of mindlessness or make less mindful choices, practice self-forgiveness and return to mindfulness.

Step 12: Ongoing Learning - Continue to deepen your understanding of mindful eating. Read books, articles, or join mindfulness communities to stay inspired and connected on your journey.

Step 13: Gratitude - Cultivate a sense of gratitude for the transformation mindful eating has brought to your life. Recognize the positive changes in your relationship with food and your overall well-being.

Step 14: Share Your Journey - Share your mindful eating journey with others. Your experiences and insights can inspire and support those around you, creating a ripple effect of mindfulness.

Step 15: Mindful Reflection - Periodically reflect on your mindful eating journey. Celebrate your progress and acknowledge the ongoing growth and evolution of your relationship with food.

By incorporating these steps into your daily life, you'll create a sustainable and fulfilling mindful eating practice. Remember that mindfulness is not a destination but a lifelong journey, and each moment is an opportunity to nurture a healthier, more mindful relationship with food and yourself. Enjoy the continued exploration and growth on this transformative path.

Overcoming Obstacles on Your Mindful Eating Journey

"As you embark on your mindful eating journey, it's important to acknowledge that obstacles may arise along the way. However, with the right strategies and a commitment to your well-being, you can overcome these challenges. Let's explore some common obstacles and how to navigate them effectively."

Time Constraints:

- *Obstacle:* In today's fast-paced world, finding time for mindful eating can be a challenge.
- *Strategy:* Prioritize self-care by allocating time for meals without distractions. Even a few minutes of mindfulness can make a significant difference.

Social Pressure:

- *Obstacle:* Social gatherings and peer pressure can lead to mindless eating.

- *Strategy:* Communicate your mindful eating goals with friends and family. Seek support from like-minded individuals who value mindfulness.

Emotional Eating:

- *Obstacle:* Emotional triggers can lead to overeating or unhealthy food choices.
- *Strategy:* Develop healthy coping mechanisms for emotions, such as journaling, meditation, or seeking support from a therapist or counselor.

Unconscious Habits:

- *Obstacle:* Mindless eating habits are deeply ingrained.
- *Strategy:* Practice self-awareness. Pause before eating and ask yourself if you're truly hungry or if you're eating out of habit or emotion.

Food Cravings:

- *Obstacle:* Strong cravings for unhealthy foods can be challenging to resist.
- *Strategy:* Acknowledge cravings without judgment. Explore healthier alternatives or allow yourself a small portion mindfully.

Limited Food Choices:

- *Obstacle:* Limited access to healthy foods can hinder mindful eating.
- *Strategy:* Opt for the healthiest options available and make the best choices within your circumstances. Advocate for improved food access in your community.

Stress and Anxiety:

- *Obstacle:* Stress and anxiety can lead to mindless snacking or overeating.

- *Strategy:* Incorporate stress-reduction practices like deep breathing, meditation, or yoga into your daily routine to manage emotional eating triggers.

Lack of Support:

- *Obstacle:* Without support from friends or family, maintaining mindfulness can be challenging.
- *Strategy:* Seek out mindfulness communities, online forums, or local groups where you can connect with others who share your goals.

Perfectionism:

- *Obstacle:* Striving for perfection in mindful eating can lead to self-criticism.
- *Strategy:* Embrace imperfection and self-compassion. Remember that mindful eating is a journey, and setbacks are part of the process.

Cultural or Social Norms: - *Obstacle:* Cultural or social norms may encourage overindulgence or mindless eating. - *Strategy:* Find ways to honor your cultural traditions while incorporating mindful eating principles. Educate others about the benefits of mindfulness.

Weight Concerns: - *Obstacle:* Fears about weight gain can deter mindful eating efforts. - *Strategy:* Focus on the holistic benefits of mindful eating, including improved well-being, rather than solely on weight-related outcomes.

Binge Eating or Disordered Eating: - *Obstacle:* Individuals with binge eating or disordered eating patterns may require specialized support. - *Strategy:* Seek guidance from a healthcare professional or therapist who specializes in eating disorders. Mindful eating can complement therapy.

Remember that obstacles are a natural part of any journey, and they provide opportunities for growth and learning. Approach your mindful eating journey with patience and self-compassion. Each challenge you overcome brings you closer to a healthier, more mindful relationship with food and yourself.

A Commitment to a Lifelong Journey

"As we conclude this mindful eating journey together, we want to extend our heartfelt congratulations to you. You've delved deep into the practice of mindfulness, transformed your relationship with food, and embarked on a path of self-discovery and well-being. But remember, this journey doesn't have an endpoint—it's a lifelong commitment to yourself and your health."

Embracing the Continual Path of Mindful Eating

"Mindful eating is not a destination; it's a way of life. It's about recognizing that every meal, every snack, every moment of nourishment is an opportunity to connect with yourself and the world around you. It's a practice that evolves with you, adapting to the changing seasons of your life."

The Gift of Self-Compassion

"As you continue your mindful eating journey, we encourage you to embrace self-compassion. Be kind to yourself, especially during moments of mindlessness or challenges. Remember that imperfection is part of being human, and each step forward is a victory worth celebrating."

Recommended Resources for Ongoing Support

"To support you on this lifelong journey, we've curated a list of recommended resources. These books, websites, and communities provide a wealth of knowledge and inspiration. Explore them to deepen your understanding of mindfulness and mindful eating."

A Motivational Speech to You, the Reader

"Dear reader, as you close this book and step into the world, we want you to carry the wisdom of mindful eating with you. This practice is not just about transforming your relationship with food; it's about transforming your relationship

with yourself. It's about recognizing your worthiness of nourishment, self-care, and a life lived with intention."

"In a world that often pulls us in a hundred different directions, mindful eating offers you a precious gift—the gift of presence. With each mindful bite, you have the opportunity to savor the beauty of the moment, to honor your body's needs, and to nourish your soul."

"You have the power to make choices that align with your well-being, choices that reflect love and respect for yourself. Remember that you are not alone on this journey. There's a community of mindful eaters around the world, each striving to live with intention and awareness."

"So, as you step forward, make this commitment to yourself: I am worthy of mindfulness, of nourishment, and of a life well-lived. Embrace each mindful meal as a moment of self-love, and let the practice of mindful eating be a guiding light on your path to greater health, happiness, and fulfillment."

"Thank you for allowing us to be a part of your journey. May your mindful eating practice continue to flourish, and may you find joy and nourishment in every mindful bite. Your journey is just beginning, and the possibilities are endless."

"With deepest gratitude and warmest wishes,

- Gabriella Goldberger

Commit to Yourself, Embrace Mindful Eating, and Live with Intention

And so, dear reader, the choice is yours—to embrace the lifelong journey of mindful eating, to savor each moment, and to honor yourself with each mindful bite. The practice of mindfulness will continue to guide you, supporting your well-being and transforming your life in ways both seen and unseen. Commit to yourself, nurture your relationship with food, and live each day with intention and presence. Your journey is a beautiful one, and it's just beginning.

Don't miss out!

Visit the website below and you can sign up to receive emails whenever Gabriella Goldberger publishes a new book. There's no charge and no obligation.

https://books2read.com/r/B-A-CNJAB-MMVNC

BOOKS 2 READ

Connecting independent readers to independent writers.